BRAIN
AND
HEART

BRAIN
AND
HEART

The Triumphs and Struggles
of a Pediatric Neurosurgeon

David I. Sandberg, M.D.
FOREWORD BY ARIANNA HUFFINGTON

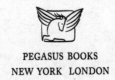

PEGASUS BOOKS
NEW YORK LONDON

BRAIN AND HEART

Pegasus Books, Ltd.
148 West 37th Street, 13th Floor
New York, NY 10018

First Pegasus Books cloth edition May 2025

Interior design by Maria Fernandez

Library of Congress Cataloging-in-Publication Data is available.

ISBN: 978-1-63936-893-8

10 9 8 7 6 5 4 3 2 1

Printed in the United States of America
Distributed by Simon & Schuster
www.pegasusbooks.com

To Mom and Dad
for your unconditional love and
guidance throughout my life

To Amy, Dalia, and Ben
for supporting me and loving me every single
day and especially on the hard days

And to my brave patients and their amazing families
for inspiring me every day with your courage

Contents

Foreword

by Arianna Huffington

The title of this book couldn't be more apt for what you'll encounter in the pages ahead. As you'll find out, there are no stories in this book about the brain that don't involve equal contributions from the heart. And that's because David Sandberg is as gifted a storyteller as he is a neurosurgeon.

As he writes, "performing surgery on the brain is unique. The brain not only controls the rest of the body, but it is also where our consciousness lives." But it's not where our full humanity lives. Drawing on his work as a pediatric neurosurgeon, Sandberg takes us inside many operating rooms, deftly explaining the high-stakes situations at hand. But he also emphasizes that many of his most meaningful moments take place outside the operating room, in clinics where he sees patients—as young as eight days old—before and after surgery, in emergency rooms where harrowing life-and-death decisions have to be made, and, especially, in communicating and connecting with families who are in the darkest moments of their lives regarding what they hold most precious: their children. Brain and heart. Life and death. Those are the stakes in all of these stories.

You don't have to be a neurosurgeon to be humbled by the brain—an organ that, as Sandberg writes, "is infinitely complicated yet also unpredictable." And you don't have to be a doctor or a patient to be profoundly moved by Sandberg's stories. Hope, loss, joy, heartbreak, grief—as Sandberg shows, these are all part of an average day for a neurosurgeon. But they are also qualities essential in all our lives, and reading this book puts them into stark relief.

Of course, Sandberg isn't just a neurosurgeon, but a pediatric neurosurgeon. In chapter 3, he writes about helping families process the "unthinkable"—a fatal diagnosis, or that their child didn't make it. "Parents' worst fears are realized when they hear me utter dreaded words— 'Your child has a brain tumor,'" he writes. Sandberg tells the story of a three-year-old named Diego, who was diagnosed with a malignant brain tumor that couldn't be operated on. Nor would chemotherapy work. Radiation could be used, but that would only prolong life for a few months, which would be miserable. After hearing this grim news,

Diego's parents, after a day of reflection and prayer, tell Sandberg they've elected to forgo treatment and take Diego home. Sandberg expresses his sorrow, hugs them, tells them what great parents they are, and then, as he says he's done many times in his career, "went home and hugged my own kids a little longer than I had the day before." And after reading this book, you will, too. And if you're not a parent, you'll have the impulse to hug those closest to you. Life for neurosurgery patients in the emergency room and on the operating table is very fragile. But it's always very fragile, for all of us, even if we take it for granted.

In fact, the lessons of *Brain and Heart* are universal and deeply relevant to all our ordinary lives. There are plenty of triumphs, like the story of Marcela, an eight-year-old from Honduras, which has many twists and turns before its unlikely and exhilarating conclusion. But it also hinges on a few pieces of luck so remarkable that the relief is tinged with thoughts of all the other children who weren't fortunate enough to cross paths with Sandberg.

In pediatric neurosurgery, as in life, there is good news and there is bad news. For the latter, in those hard conversations with parents, Sandberg writes that he focuses on three key components: compassion, honesty, and listening. That's a good guide for any meaningful conversation. When receiving bad news, Sandberg recounts, parents react in all sorts of ways: rage, denial, wailing, and silence. And each of these is deeply human and valid—there is no "right" way to process life's most difficult challenges.

Sandberg also writes about work-life balance. Being on call as a surgeon often means demanding hours—as does the training in residency, when one hundred–hour weeks are common. He notes that the divorce rate at one neurosurgery residency program was over 100 percent—because some residents actually got divorced twice. But at the same time, Sandberg writes that he has never missed a family birthday or important event: "I encourage medical students considering a career in neurosurgery to understand the challenges of this road but to also know that it is possible to be a neurosurgeon and still have a wonderful family life."

Prediction: You will come away from *Brain and Heart* with a greater appreciation of safety. If your children don't wear a bike helmet now, they will after this book. Likewise, you'll feel a sense of outrage at our gun laws after seeing the horrific downstream consequences through the eyes of a pediatric neurosurgeon. The book is also eye-opening about the issue of health equity, with some of the most heart-warming and heartrending stories coming from Sandberg's humanitarian relief missions to places like Guatemala, Mexico, Haiti, Peru, and Uganda.

A word of warning, however. Though this book is hard to put down, I would caution against reading it in public, as you will likely burst into tears regularly. Some of those will be tears of sadness, and some will also be tears of joy. And because of the aforementioned unpredictability of the brain, one can change to the other very suddenly.

Most of all, what comes through is Sandberg's heart. As he shares, he didn't plan on becoming a neurosurgeon—in many ways, neurosurgery seems to have chosen him. And we can all be thankful for that. What these stories lay bare aren't just the riveting medical mysteries of the brain, but our essential humanity, and what really matters when everything else is stripped away. Sandberg writes that he's come away with a better appreciation of a saying from the Talmud that his parents taught him growing up: "A person who saves one life is as if he saved a whole world." We can't all save lives in this way, but we can all make a difference to those around us. And you'll be inspired to after reading this book.

Introduction

I remember the very first moment I saw and touched a human brain. The exhilaration of opening up a skull and seeing the brain pulsating with every heartbeat is hard to describe. Knowing that the tissue I was looking at controls the amazingly complex functions of thinking, feeling, talking, seeing, remembering, and performing complex motor tasks—all that makes us human—blew me away. Almost thirty years later, the experience remains just as profound.

The allure of performing surgeries is only one component of the day-to-day experience of being a brain and spine surgeon for children. Many of my most meaningful experiences take place in the outpatient clinic, emergency room, or surgical waiting area where I communicate with families. In these locations, on so many occasions, I need to take a deep breath before walking into a room, sitting down, and having one of the most important conversations in the entire lives of those families. Before entering that room, I need to put aside everything else going through my mind—other patients I am caring for, other families or doctors waiting to speak to me, emails and phone calls waiting to be returned, things going on with my own family—and fully focus on the critical task at hand. I am aware that the conversation I am about to have will be remembered for the rest of their lives. Every facial expression I make and every word I choose may be critically important in guiding life-changing decisions.

On some days, I am the bearer of the very worst news imaginable to parents—that a child has died or has no hope of surviving a devastating car accident or a gunshot wound to the head or spontaneous bleeding in the brain. I have told parents that their child may live but will never walk or talk again. Parents' worst fears are realized when they hear me utter dreaded words—"Your child has a brain tumor." Sometimes I have to give parents this news at the same moment as additional tragedies are occurring, such as the death of another family member in the same car accident or while another immediate family member is also dying of cancer. As a parent whose children are my whole world, I recognize how crushing my words are to these parents.

These conversations are never easy. In fact, many doctors choose non-pediatric specialties to avoid giving bad news about children. On the other hand, I also have the great joy of celebrating the most wonderful news with parents—that their child has made a remarkable recovery after a serious surgery or is cured of her brain tumor and will live a normal life. In fact, I give good news much more often than bad news, and these conversations are rewarding beyond measure. In a single day at work, I often experience a roller coaster of emotions—sharing the worst devastation with some families and the greatest exhilaration or relief with others.

Sometimes I face the challenge of helping parents make difficult choices about their child's health when critical decisions are not black and white. All surgeries have risks and benefits, and existing medical knowledge has not defined the best path forward in all situations. In many cases, there is no perfect choice, and parents must choose between two bad options. For example, they might have to choose between waiting to see if a benign brain tumor will grow on its own and cause loss of a patient's hand function versus undergoing a surgery that has a five percent chance of causing an immediate and devastating loss of this same function. The hardest part is that, so often, there isn't an obviously correct decision, and the parents will never know the outcome of the opposite choice.

In each of these conversations, I recognize that every word I say is important, and I choose each one carefully. I try to be as compassionate as possible while being completely honest. It has often struck me that, during these conversations, parents hang on to my every word and try to process what I am saying but have no idea what is actually going through my mind. The purpose of this memoir of my life as a pediatric neurosurgeon is to openly share what I am thinking and feeling during each of these conversations. In the pages that follow, I tell the stories of patients who have changed my life and the joy, heartbreak, uncertainty, and physical and emotional challenges that come with performing brain surgery on children. I bare my soul, sharing with readers something they otherwise would never have access to—my private thoughts when I make the most complex choices that change the lives of my patients and their families forever. The reader will understand not only the demands and rewards of being a pediatric neurosurgeon, but also what I go through emotionally when I make agonizing decisions or give parents the worst news imaginable.

Why do I want to share my innermost thoughts and feelings when having a difficult or emotional conversation? First and most important, I think that it would greatly benefit families to understand what is going through the mind of their child's doctor during these moments. I want families to know the truth—that even the most experienced doctors have fears and insecurities and sometimes make mistakes. I want families to understand the context of my thought processes by knowing what I went through during my training and what a day in my life is like. I want families to know what keeps me awake at night.

I want families to know how I emotionally process unpredictable outcomes, devastating surgical complications, preventable tragedies, and fatal diagnoses. My hope is that this knowledge will lead to greater overall understanding of their loved one's condition and helps them navigate the great challenges they face.

As an academician who trains the next generation of surgeons, I also wrote this book for medical students and trainees, particularly in surgical subspecialties. I hope that by reading this book, young physicians and future physicians will learn from my experience how to make interactions with families as positive as possible without sacrificing honesty. I hope that young physicians and surgeons will understand that they are not alone when they struggle to process the implications of bad outcomes and surgical complications. I am hopeful that medical trainees interested in clinical research will learn from my experiences as I have tried to develop new treatment options for a fatal disease. Finally, I share my thoughts on medical care in low- and middle-income countries based upon my many experiences volunteering abroad, and I explain how these experiences have shaped my worldview.

In describing what goes through my mind in the many situations I encounter, I often do so through the medium of sharing stories about patients. In some of these stories, I include patients' real names. Of course, this is done with the permission of their parents and/or the patients themselves if age appropriate. In other stories, based upon the families' request or my own judgment, I use a pseudonym. In all cases, whether I use real names or pseudonyms, I tell these stories honestly and without embellishment. I do so with the utmost admiration for my brave patients and their incredible parents who are struggling to make impossible decisions and process news that no parent should ever have to hear. I also do so with the most profound gratitude to these parents who place their trust in me to care for their precious children.

No medical specialty requires more intense training than neurosurgery. The profession is grueling and exhilarating in equal measure. Neurosurgeons are a small cadre of physicians entrusted to operate on the most complicated structure in the human body, yet *Brain and Heart* is a memoir that acknowledges the humility that comes with performing surgery on the brain. Even the best training and the most modern technology have limits in the face of the challenging diseases I treat. Trying to save the lives of children who have been injured by car accidents or gunshot wounds, brain tumors, or other devastating conditions is a highly imperfect science. In so many circumstances when treating these conditions, not all choices are clear. Sometimes the correct decision cannot be made based only upon existing medical literature, many years of experience, or discussing a case with colleagues. I have learned time and time again that my profession requires not only my brain, but my heart as well.

1

When the Brain Humbles You: Facing Unpredictable Outcomes

O n May 31, 2017, Garrett was a perfectly healthy fifteen-year-old boy when he rolled out of bed. Just a few hours later, Garrett was on the brink of death. In fact, Garrett was as close to being brain-dead as you can be without actually meeting formal brain death criteria. It was up to me to decide whether to offer an operation that could potentially save his life. It wasn't a straightforward decision.

As the pediatric neurosurgeon on call that day at Children's Memorial Hermann Hospital in Houston, I had received a call that a patient was being "life-flighted" in. Life Flight is the hospital's emergency helicopter transport system that provides rapid transport for the sickest patients who are transferred to our center from other locations in Houston and beyond. I was asked: Do you accept the patient? This is a formality. The answer is always yes. I was given the patient's estimated time of arrival at the hospital; Garrett was only twelve minutes away. I rushed to the Emergency Department (ED) to be there when he arrived.

Garrett had suffered a severe traumatic head injury. He was riding on the back of a friend's ATV in a community fifty miles south of Houston when he was thrown from the four-wheeler and hit his head on the asphalt. A CT scan of Garrett's brain showed a large epidural hematoma—a blood clot between the skull and the thick, leathery covering of the brain called the dura mater. The skull protects the brain's delicate tissue but also limits how much space there is for the brain to swell or move. As a result, when an epidural hematoma shifts the brain from one side to another, important brain structures can be damaged or destroyed very quickly. In Garrett's case, the CT scan showed that the blood clot was pushing the left side of his brain inward toward the right. When the brain is compressed in this manner, from the outside toward the inside, the results can be catastrophic.

In fact, Garrett almost didn't even make it to the hospital. He was unconscious at the scene of the accident for about thirty minutes before paramedics arrived. The paramedics quickly called the Children's Memorial Hermann Hospital Life Flight air ambulance team, which arrived

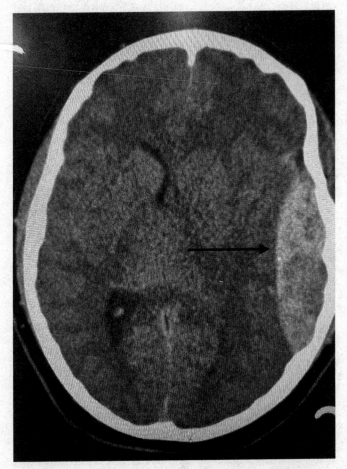

Figure 1. *Garrett's CT scan showing epidural blood clot, marked by arrow. The blood clot is shifting the brain from left to right (the left side of the brain is the right side of the image).*

minutes later. A paramedic placed a breathing tube in order to protect Garrett's airway and make sure his lungs received enough oxygen. Garrett was then loaded onto the helicopter for the quick flight to the hospital. However, there was a delay. The helicopter couldn't take off because Garrett's heart rate was extremely low—under forty beats per minute—and protocols required a heart rate of at least forty for the flight to take off.

The protocols are in place so the Life Flight team does not transport a patient who dies en route to the hospital. They also don't want to be performing CPR in flight. The reason for Garrett's low heart rate was increased pressure in the brain caused by the blood clot. When pressure in the brain is so high that it triggers the heart rate to drop, this is a sign that the patient is in imminent danger of devastating damage to the brain or rapid progression to brain death. Luckily for Garrett, the delay was brief. When his heartbeat rose above forty, the helicopter took off.

As I stood next to the unconscious teenager, I first had to make sure Garrett was not brain-dead. Brain death occurs when the heart continues to beat but no brain function can be demonstrated in a bedside examination. To reach a determination of brain death for Garrett, I needed to find that his breathing could only be maintained by a ventilator, that he was unconscious and unresponsive to painful stimulation, and that various bedside tests of his cranial nerves yielded no signs of brain stem function. In physiological terms, brain death means that the brain stem has undergone catastrophic and irreversible damage. In the United States, if a patient is declared brain-dead, this is considered the equivalent of being declared dead, and he or she is then removed from life support.

The brain stem is the most primitive part of the brain, sitting at the base of the brain just above the spine. The brain stem is responsible for such basic functions as breathing, blood pressure, and heart rate. It is also incredibly sensitive. That's why some tumors within the brain stem are inoperable. Even the slightest insult can result in a catastrophic injury or death. A blood clot like Garrett's, which compressed his brain into a smaller space, puts pressure on his brain stem. I needed to find out whether that pressure had already left the teenager brain-dead.

First, I checked whether Garrett was breathing above the ventilator. The machine was giving him twelve breaths per minute. If Garrett was breathing at all on his own, he would be taking thirteen or fourteen breaths per minute or more. That would be a sign of brain stem activity. Unfortunately, Garrett was not. Only the ventilator was keeping him alive.

With a sinking feeling, I began the neurological exam. As his father, Kurt, looked on, I opened Garrett's eyelids to look at his pupils. They were larger than normal and did not react when I shined a flashlight in his eyes. "Blown pupils" was a sign that pressure from the blood clot had compromised Garrett's brain stem. Unreactive pupils are used as a proxy for the brain stem because the nerve that controls the pupils, the oculomotor (third) cranial nerve, sits next to the brain stem. Damage to this nerve causes one or both pupils to dilate. When neither of Garrett's pupils became smaller when I shined the flashlight into his eyes, this meant that the blood clot was compressing the brain enough to affect the oculomotor nerve. It was also a sign of a likely injury to the neighboring brain stem. Unresponsive pupils by themselves are not enough to declare brain death. Nonetheless, this was a very bad sign. If Garrett was not already brain-dead, this was a sign he soon would be.

I then tested Garrett's corneal blink reflex by touching the surface of each eye with a piece of gauze. He did not blink. Like the pupils, blinking is one of the most basic, natural responses. The corneal blink reflex test assesses the integrity of two other cranial nerves, the trigeminal (fifth) nerve and the facial (seventh) nerve. Even people with a rare condition called "locked-in syndrome," who are unable to speak or move any other part of their body, are still able to blink. Garrett's inability to blink when his corneal blink reflex was tested was another sign that his brain stem was not functioning normally.

I pressed my pen into Garrett's fingernails—a very painful maneuver—and he did not respond. I tried a sternal rub, pushing very hard on Garrett's chest with my fist, and he did not flinch. Like reacting to light or blinking, reacting to pain is a fundamental human response. Four times, I pinched his trapezius muscles—the muscles between his neck and shoulder—extremely hard. He did not move at all. With even minimal brain function, a painful stimulus like this should provoke some sort of reaction. Even a flicker of movement would be something. Garrett remained motionless.

I was about to give up and tell Kurt that his son's life could not be saved when I decided to pinch Garrett one more time as hard as I could. With that last pinch, Garrett had a response called extensor posturing. He extended his arms just slightly. While better than no response at all, this was certainly not a reason for optimism. Extensor posturing typically signifies a severe and often irreversible injury to the brain stem. In other words, Garrett was alive but just barely. And now I had to decide what to do. Should I operate or not? The decision had to be made immediately, as the only possible way to save a patient's life in this circumstance is to remove the blood clot right away. If the blood clot was not removed, Garrett faced certain death.

By the time Garrett arrived in the Emergency Department, I had more than a decade of experience as an attending pediatric neurosurgeon in addition to my seven years of intense residency and fellowship training. Garrett's neurological examination was so poor that I considered a good outcome extremely unlikely. I thought of the many hundreds of children I had cared for over the years with severe traumatic brain injuries. Children can surprise us with unexpectedly good outcomes at times, but Garrett's neurological examination, especially with large, unreactive pupils, told me the great likelihood was that—even with surgery—Garrett would either progress to brain death or have a devastating outcome, such as being nonverbal and bedridden for the rest of his life. I had never seen a good outcome in a child with a neurological examination as poor as Garrett's. I thought to myself that if Garrett were my child, I would request that nothing should be done at this point. In these terrible moments, doctors must help parents make quick decisions that have implications for their child and their family for years to come.

I am reminded of the long-term implications of these choices every time I see another patient, a seventeen-year-old boy named Nathan, for whom I have cared for years. Nathan was born prematurely, and his first APGAR score was just two. APGAR scores are given by healthcare professionals right after birth and are the very first assessment of a baby's health. An acronym for Appearance, Pulse, Grimace, Activity, and Respiration, APGAR scores range from one to ten, with two being a terrible score. Nathan needed a breathing tube placed shortly after birth. Despite the breathing tube, he suffered severe damage to his brain, which did not receive enough oxygen at some point during the birthing process. His parents, although informed of his poor prognosis, were hoping for a miracle, and at every point in time, they chose to pursue any intervention that would keep him alive.

I became involved in Nathan's care in order to treat his hydrocephalus, a condition in which the fluid produced by the brain does not circulate properly. Intervention is needed to maintain normal pressure in the brain. For Nathan, I placed a shunt to drain fluid from the head to the abdomen and thereby relieve pressure in the brain. Shunts can be lifesaving devices for many children, but they can also be associated with many complications. Like a car or an air conditioner, shunts can work for years and then fail without warning. When they fail, patients can become very sick due to increased pressure in the brain. Periodically, Nathan comes to the hospital for evaluation when there is suspicion that his shunt may not be working. He is very difficult to evaluate because he is so neurologically devastated. He has never walked or spoken a single word. He lies in bed, and his limbs are very stiff. He is fed by a gastric tube, more commonly called a "G-tube"—a feeding tube through which liquid nutrition is administered because he cannot eat. The only sounds he makes are grunting noises. He does not follow commands like squeezing a hand or opening his eyes when asked to do so, and he likely doesn't understand any words that are spoken to him.

Each time Nathan gets admitted to the hospital, I wonder to myself whether Nathan's parents knew what they were signing up for when they chose to pursue intervention after intervention that kept him alive since infancy—and do they regret those decisions? I have never asked his mother this question, but I think I know the answer based upon her actions. Every time she brings Nathan to the hospital, she is there day and night, often up all night, and never leaves his bedside. She is so upset when she thinks Nathan is in pain. Her love for Nathan is awe-inspiring to me, because when I am honest with myself I don't know if I could make the same sacrifices she has made if I had been in her shoes. I think to myself that, if my own child laid in bed all day and had never run into my arms or uttered a word or understood me, I would not be able to give as much love and devotion as Nathan's mother. And she is not alone. There are many mothers and fathers and grandparents of neurologically devastated children I have encountered who demonstrate similar love and sacrifice year after year. These parents have my profound admiration, as I recognize that they have a rare and extraordinary inner strength.

I did my best to explain Garrett's situation to his parents. I did so realizing how difficult it was for them to envision what a poor outcome looks like for their child, especially what a poor outcome looks like in five years or twenty years. Would they want him to live if his life would be like Nathan's? Picturing a once-vibrant child living as an unresponsive or uncomprehending adult is an almost impossible task. Parents facing the sudden loss of a child have a hard enough time thinking about the next hour or the next day. They have been crushed by a moment more terrible than anything they could have ever imagined. Given circumstances like Garrett's, almost all parents will ask me to do anything I can to save their child, no matter what the odds.

As I considered whether to operate, I also thought briefly about our department's Morbidity and Mortality conference, more commonly called "M&M." M&M is a surgeons-only gathering where we present cases to our colleagues in a formal setting to discuss situations in which patients die or have complications. If Garrett died on the operating room table or soon afterward, my judgment to operate on someone as close to death as Garrett would be called into question. I knew some of my colleagues would ask why I operated on a patient with dilated pupils who was nearly brain-dead. When a patient's neurological examination is so poor, some would assert that offering surgery deviates from what is considered "standard of care." I also knew that deaths soon after surgery were harmful to statistics on operative mortality that are tracked by our department. These were all fleeting thoughts. Having to present my case at M&M does not actually deter me at all. I decided long ago that I am willing to face the judgment of my colleagues if there might be a chance to save a child.

Performing surgery on the brain is unique. The brain not only controls the rest of the body, but it is also where our consciousness lives. It houses our memories and our personality. The brain is infinitely complicated, yet it is also unpredictable. The brain is not a computer or a car engine that can be run through determinative diagnostic tests. How the brain responds to injury is elusive and hard to assess, especially in children. As a general rule, the younger the child, the more unpredictable the brain's response to surgery. That's because a child's brain is sometimes capable of remodeling itself, even after terrible injuries. In a very young child, a neurosurgeon can remove half of the brain and the child is sometimes able to compensate. For example, when parts of the brain normally devoted to language are injured, language function can sometimes shift to the opposite side of the brain. The brains of children can remake themselves in other amazing ways after they are damaged by bleeding or partially removed during surgery. That's why Garrett's case was so difficult. Even though I had never seen a great outcome in someone with a neurological examination as poor as Garrett's, I could not say with certainty that surgery would not help. If Garrett were an old man instead of a healthy teenager, I would have been more certain that he would have no chance of meaningful survival. But because a child's brain is capable of remarkable resilience, there were no such certainties in Garrett's case. Accepting uncertainty comes with being a pediatric neurosurgeon.

While uncertainty can lead to indecision, there was no time to mull over this choice. Every minute counted. How quickly a trauma patient gets from the Emergency Department to the operating room can mean the difference between life and death. At Children's Memorial Hermann Hospital, the time from arrival to the operating room is often less than ten minutes. The average time from arrival to skin incision is under forty minutes. Hospitals keep track of these statistics because time is so important.

I looked over at Garrett's dad. I needed to make a decision immediately. I explained Garrett's neurological status and the likelihood that even if he survived, Garrett would not be the same kid that his father knew and loved. I tried to do so with kindness and compassion, but I was brutally honest. Conversations like these are often the single worst moments of a parent's life. Kurt was clearly devastated, but he was quite composed. He is a big, strong man—a former professional baseball player, I later learned. But he has a gentle manner, and I remember thinking to myself that I like this guy.

I asked Kurt whether he had other children. In retrospect, I have no idea why I asked this question, as it is not part of my usual routine. And, in truth, this is completely irrelevant. Whether Garrett was Kurt's only child or if he had ten others should have no bearing on this decision. Kurt answered in a soft but definitive voice that Garrett was his only child, and he asked me again to take him to surgery if there was even the smallest chance his son would survive. Minutes later, Garrett's mom, Holly, arrived. There was no time for another discussion, as the operating room was ready, and it was now or never. I briefly explained the situation to Holly, who also agreed that we should operate, and then I raced to the operating room with Garrett.

I performed a hemicraniectomy on Garrett, removing the left side of his skull, and I immediately encountered a large blood clot as expected. I removed the blood clot and placed a small electrode into the frontal lobe of Garrett's brain so that we could monitor the pressure in his brain after surgery. I closed his scalp, leaving the bone off so that the brain had room for the expected subsequent swelling. I thought to myself that we should only be so lucky to put this kid's bone back on with another operation down the road. We took Garrett to the pediatric intensive care unit and obtained a postoperative CT scan that showed evacuation of the blood clot and improvement of the midline shift that was present before the operation.

Garrett's parents prayed that he would wake up, but based upon my past experience, I had little hope that he would do so. I was just grateful that he had not died on the operating room table. To my surprise and delight, immediately after surgery, Garrett's pupils were normal in size and reacted appropriately when we shined a flashlight. Soon afterward, he began purposefully moving his arms and legs. Over the next few days, as his sedation was weaned, he began to follow commands, squeezing my hands or wiggling his toes when asked to do so. The pressure in his brain was normal, so we removed both his breathing tube and intracranial pressure monitor on the third day after surgery. Soon after the breathing tube came out, he recognized his parents and began to talk coherently.

Garrett improved every single day. Ten days after his admission, he was transferred to an inpatient rehabilitation unit, and we later replaced the part of his skull that had been removed. Against all odds, he made a complete

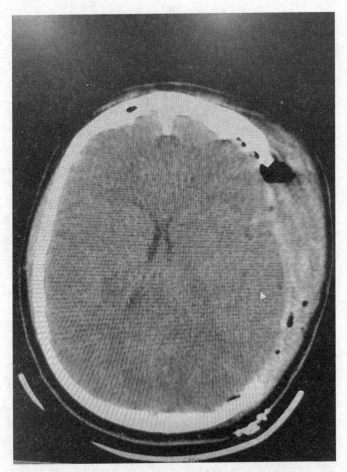

Figure 2. *CT scan after Garrett's surgery showing that the blood clot has been removed and the brain is no longer shifted. A hemicraniectomy (removal of a large portion of one side of the skull) has been performed.*

recovery. Later that year, Garrett went back to school. He graduated from high school, where he played on the golf team. After high school, he studied nuclear power, and he recently started a job at a nuclear power plant. If you saw him or spoke to him, you would never know that he had been on the brink of death. He is 100 percent neurologically normal, just as he was before the accident. Garrett's outcome was beyond what I could have imagined in my wildest dreams. Not only had his life been saved, but he was the same person he was before his accident.

To Garrett's parents and to me, his complete recovery is nothing short of a miracle. Kurt and Holly are wonderful and loving people, and they have become dear friends. Their gratitude is limitless. Over the years since his injury, they have showered me and my team of physician assistants and medical assistants with generous gifts, and most important, with their love. And yet, despite this happy ending, Garrett's case haunts me. Since Garrett's injury, I have reviewed his situation in my mind countless times. While I ultimately took Garrett to the operating room and saved his life, I came very close to not doing so. What would have happened if I hadn't pinched Garrett that one last time? With no brain stem responses at all, I would not have offered surgery, and Garrett would be dead. To do otherwise would have deviated from the standard of care. Were there other kids who might have had minimal signs of brain stem function that were only apparent on the third or fourth or fifth neurological examination whose lives may have been saved if only I had offered surgery? I have racked my brain, and I can't think of any specific cases, but it is certainly possible that they exist.

I have learned over the years that doctors are often inaccurate in forecasting outcomes. Understandably, this can be extremely frustrating to parents. When a patient is diagnosed with a fatal disease, a loved one will ask how much time they have left. This is such a basic and important question, yet the answers we give are often wrong. In a study of terminally ill patients, doctors' predictions were accurate (within 33 percent of actual survival) only one in five times.[1] My colleagues and I are also often wrong when predicting the extent of recovery when a patient has a new neurological problem from an injury, stroke, or surgery. I can do the same exact operation on two kids, removing a tumor from the same region of the brain. The operations can appear identical in every way, yet one kid wakes up perfectly normal and the other wakes up with new neurological problems. We are wrong in both directions. Sometimes we are too optimistic, perhaps because we are so hopeful that a patient will recover. Other times, as in Garrett's case, we are too pessimistic. In the years since Garrett's injury, his case comes to mind every single time I see a child with a severe traumatic brain injury and a poor neurological examination. I still have the same grim conversation with families in which I honestly explain the likelihood of death or severe disability, but I think of Garrett—and I know that there is a flicker of hope.

Not a single child I have cared for since Garrett has made as dramatic a recovery as he did with such a poor preoperative neurological examination. Other children have either died or have a range of disabilities, often quite severe. Some cannot walk, talk, or interact with their families. Many of them lie in bed all day, fed by tubes, and I wonder if their parents regret agreeing to surgery. My own children are my whole world, and yet when I am honest with myself, I know that for me, I would choose death for them over this outcome if it could be predicted with certainty. I suspect that many other parents would, too. But, when faced with the decision of whether or not to operate in a moment of crisis, nearly all parents ask me to try to save their child's life. It is simply impossible for parents to assess the implications of this choice clearly in the moment. Parents whose love for their child is immeasurable will often, understandably, cling to any flicker of hope until their child's last breath. Hope is not rational but rather is a truly human emotion that is hard to supersede.

There is an old, disparaging joke about neurosurgeons. "What's the difference between God and a neurosurgeon?" The answer: "God doesn't think he's a neurosurgeon." In contrast, I have learned throughout my career that neurosurgery is quite a humbling profession. We are human, and all humans are sometimes mistaken in their judgment. Each of us can take great pride in the lives we have saved or improved, but we also must live with the mistakes we have made—or almost made in Garrett's case—that have life-and-death implications with the potential to devastate families. Even though performing neurosurgery on children requires great confidence in one's abilities, it also requires an acceptance of the limits of our knowledge about the human brain and our ability to treat it. It also requires a recognition of the tremendous power of the uniquely human emotion of hope that makes us all cling to any possibility that our loved ones can be saved when tragedy strikes.

A Tough Road:
The Making of a Pediatric
Neurosurgeon

S ome individuals decide to become neurosurgeons right out of the womb. I am not one of them. My journey to neurosurgery—and then pediatric neurosurgery— was a long and complex one and involved a certain amount of serendipity. I did know that I wanted to be a doctor from a very young age. Like many boys, I admired my father and wanted to be just like him when I grew up. I also increasingly appreciated that he seemed to have more job satisfaction than the average grown-up. My dad is an ophthalmologist who talked frequently throughout my childhood about how much he loved his job. He loved both seeing patients in the office and performing surgeries.

He felt like he was helping people every day. He worked hard while in the office, but his hours were very reasonable and he was completely in control of his schedule. We ate dinner together every night, and my dad rarely had to see patients or perform surgeries on nights, weekends, or holidays. Throughout my childhood, he was very present in my life—he coached my childhood basketball team and was a truly engaged father. His life choices seemed to be great ones to emulate.

As a teenager, I knew absolutely nothing about neuroscience. I was mostly focused on getting good grades and succeeding in sports. In tenth grade, I faced my first major disappointment in life—the realization that despite countless hours on the basketball court throughout my childhood, I wasn't ever going to get playing time on my large public high school's team. I was too small, too slow, and simply not talented enough. I knew that the writing was on the wall when the junior varsity coach frequently bellowed during jumping drills, "Sandberg, you can only jump hamburger high!" I switched to swimming and water polo and worked hard enough to become a decent water polo player and earn a spot on my university's team. I went to college without plans to do much outside of school besides play water polo and enjoy college life.

Academically, I planned to be pre-med, primarily because I was emulating my father. My most influential medical experiences—late in high school and early in college— were tagging along with my dad on ophthalmology medical missions to the Dominican Republic, Jamaica, and Antigua. These trips opened my eyes to the great inequities in the world, as I saw so many patients who were nearly blind from easily treatable conditions such as cataracts. They made me even more attracted to the idea of becoming a doctor from the standpoint of public service, a value emphasized to my sisters and me by my parents throughout our childhood.

Soon after I got to college in Boston, I had a transformative experience. As the weather became colder, I found myself shivering each day despite the huge winter coat my parents bought for me when they dropped me off at college. As I walked to and from class, I was struck by the sight of many homeless men and women sleeping in the streets—even in sub-freezing temperatures. My shock was quite naïve, of course, but I had lived a sheltered childhood in the suburbs of Miami where I saw few homeless people and it never got so cold. I wondered why these poor men and women had nowhere to sleep besides the hard cold ground in the middle of winter. Why was this their best option? And why did they not sleep in homeless shelters? I resolved to find the answers to these questions.

I discovered that there was a homeless shelter run by students at a nearby church, and I began to volunteer there. At first, I served leftover food from the student dining hall that was delivered daily to the shelter by student volunteers. It felt good to be helping in a small way, but I was disappointed that it was hard to really get to know any of the homeless men and women as they quickly moved through the food line. I learned that the shelter had a program, run by students, in which volunteers were paired with homeless individuals who were actively trying to find jobs and then move into permanent housing. I immediately volunteered for this program. I was paired with a homeless man whom I was tasked with helping to create a résumé, obtain suitable clothes for job interviews, and apply for jobs. As I got to know this man and many other homeless individuals with whom I worked during my college years, I learned that health issues were one of the many obstacles that prevented so many people from escaping homelessness.

Some of the clients with whom I worked had mental illness or chronic diseases that made it impossible for them to keep a regular work schedule. None had health insurance. They could not afford medicines, and their only means of receiving any medical care was through emergency rooms. Many avoided even going to emergency rooms because they felt as though they were treated there with disdain. Some had wounds that were caused or worsened by poor hygiene, as daily cleanliness was hard to maintain while living on the streets without regular access to showers. My work with the homeless ingrained in me the most compelling reason for becoming a doctor, beyond just wanting to be like my dad. I could not imagine anything more meaningful than a career helping indigent patients overcome these immense challenges.

I went to medical school with the intention of becoming a primary care doctor working in an inner city with a focus on caring for underserved populations such as the homeless. During my first two years of medical school, which were largely spent in the classroom, I did take note that my favorite course was neuroscience. It blew my mind to learn how, in a matter of milliseconds, an impulse from the brain could make a person speak or wiggle their toes or process a visual image. I was also fascinated by how much was still left to learn about the brain. Scientists seemed to have pretty much figured out how the heart, lungs, liver, kidneys, and other organs performed their functions, but so much about the brain remained a mystery. Still, my most meaningful activity was volunteering to help provide medical care to the homeless, and my plans to pursue a career in primary care in an urban setting serving the needy remained unchanged.

The third year of medical school included rotations in various fields of medicine. This was my chance to sample the many career options available to doctors and decide which field of residency training to pursue. Until my neurosurgery rotation, the rotation that made the single biggest impact on me was emergency medicine. In the emergency room, patients are triaged both according to their level of severity—the sickest patients are identified to receive care rapidly—and as either "medical" or "surgical." To my surprise, I found myself gravitating toward the surgical patients, especially the ones who needed emergency interventions. It was so dramatic and exciting to watch surgeons take immediate action to save a person's life after a trauma or other critical event that required surgical intervention. I tried to get myself assigned to help care for patients triaged to surgery at every opportunity, and I realized that I needed to have an open mind and consider surgical specialties.

During my general surgery rotation, I was not overwhelmed by the surgical procedures. As a medical student, I was either not scrubbed in—standing in the corner bored out of my mind because I couldn't see anything—or scrubbed in but standing for hours in an awkward position holding a retractor and still couldn't see much. What actually made me decide to become a surgeon was not the operating room (OR) experience, but rather my time spent in clinic with surgeons. I loved the surgical approach to diseases. Typically, a patient would show up at the surgeon's office with a single, very scary problem. The surgeon would then examine the patient, review imaging findings, and tell the patient and family how he or she was going to fix the problem along with the risks and benefits of doing so. These conversations were intense and meaningful. And then, I witnessed how satisfying it was for the surgeon to fix the problem definitively and earn the eternal gratitude of patients and families. Even though the operating room wasn't much fun for me as a student, I could see that the residents and faculty loved their time spent in the OR.

As I worked with more and more doctors in different specialties, I also did some self-reflection about my own disposition and realized that my personality was more "surgical" than "medical." There are certain stereotypes regarding the personalities of various types of doctors that are overplayed and not always accurate, but have grains of truth in my assessment. Medical doctors tend to be contemplative and love to solve medical mysteries—to figure out from scratch what is wrong with patients. They have the patience to manage patients with multiple, complex medical problems. They have broad expertise about many disease processes affecting different organ systems. Surgeons, on the other hand, like to act quickly and definitively to solve a single problem. Most often, patients come to a surgeon with a diagnosis already made, and the surgeon is tasked with performing an operation to address the illness. Surgeons also, stereotypically, are sometimes reputed to be arrogant jerks. My own observation as a medical student was that this was true of only a minority of surgeons; most were actually kind and caring and highly sympathetic to the struggles of their patients. And, of course, I knew that every profession has its share of jerks. I decided to become a surgeon.

The next step was figuring out what type of surgeon to become. I decided to choose elective rotations in urology—because my medical school had a world-famous urologist, Pat Walsh, M.D., who was my assigned mentor; ophthalmology—because my dad loved it so much; and neurosurgery—because I remembered how much I had enjoyed the neuroscience course and thought it would be neat to see brain surgery. I figured that, in the end, I would probably become an ophthalmologist like my father.

My neurosurgery rotation was the last of these three, and I was absolutely blown away by the experience. First, it was immediately clear that the neurosurgery residents were among the hardest working residents in the hospital, but they were also the happiest. Unlike some residents in other specialties who seemed tired and grumpy and often complained, the neurosurgery residents worked day and night, but loved their jobs. The neurosurgery team had a certain esprit de corps that made me want to be a part of it. Every team member felt valued, and residents at all levels seemed fascinated and excited by the surgeries they were performing. And boy were these surgeries amazing! I got to scrub in on surgeries to repair skull fractures, evacuate brain hemorrhages, remove brain tumors, repair damaged nerves, and so much more. Although I worked long hours and stayed up all night helping the resident on call many nights, I was much less tired during the day than I had been on some easier rotations. I was hooked. By the end of the month, I was fairly certain that I was going to become a neurosurgeon. I canceled my scheduled elective rotations for the next four months to work in a neurosurgery research laboratory with the primary goal of making my residency application more competitive.

But doubts entered my mind. I loved my one month as a student on the neurosurgery service, but it was only a month. Would I love neurosurgery for the next thirty years or more? And particularly, would I love the lifestyle? Would the long days and late nights managing emergencies get old? Could I be a neurosurgeon and also a good husband and father like my dad? Would I be able to coach my kids' sports teams? I was taken aback when I learned that the divorce rate at one prestigious neurosurgery residency program was *over* 100 percent—because a few residents actually got divorced twice during their residency. It made me nervous to hear a joke that had some truth in it that was told about some neurosurgery residency programs: "What's the downside of being on call every other night?" The answer: "You miss half of the good cases."

Another doubt that frequently entered my mind was whether, by choosing to become a neurosurgeon, I was straying from my original goal to treat the underserved. This goal was still a very important part of my vision of what I wanted to accomplish during my career. It was problematic for me that, as a student, I encountered more opportunities to have a career focused on serving indigent patients in medical specialties than surgical ones.

My parents were surprised by my decision and questioned it. They were particularly concerned about the lifestyle of a neurosurgeon. Did I really want to choose a job in which I would be awakened by emergencies night after night and work such long hours? My father reminded me often about how much he loved his job as an ophthalmologist and how content the overwhelming majority of ophthalmologists are with their career choice. I knew that, if I completed an ophthalmology residency, I would have a great opportunity to join his successful ophthalmology practice.

The answers to my many questions about whether neurosurgery would ultimately be the right choice for me were unknown. I had real doubts, which was unfortunate because the decision was so consequential. But at the end of the day, I was stuck on the passion I felt during my neurosurgery rotation, and I knew that I needed to do something about which I was passionate. I was convinced that I would wake up each morning more excited to go to work as a neurosurgeon than any other type of doctor. I felt that I had no real choice but to follow this new dream. I decided to move forward and become a neurosurgeon, and I was so excited when I matched at an outstanding residency program in New York City.

Becoming a resident in neurosurgery is similar to enlisting in an elite military unit. When I signed up, I was well aware that I was choosing brutally long working hours, sleep deprivation, and huge personal sacrifice. And I knew that during my residency I would completely lose control over my daily life. My days would be long and stressful, often without adequate time to eat enough, let alone go to the grocery store to get something in case I had time to eat. Residents rarely have time for exercise or much else outside of the hospital. Those who have children often go days or weeks in which they barely see their kids. Why would anyone voluntarily submit to this life? I chose this road knowing not only the challenges that lay ahead but also the tremendous rewards. I knew that I was in store for an exciting and meaningful journey. My mind and my hands would meet their most compelling task—saving lives by performing the most technically challenging surgeries. Despite their physical and mental demands, neurosurgery residencies are very competitive, with many talented applicants competing for coveted positions.

When I was a resident from 1997 to 2003, the length of neurosurgery residency training in the United States varied from six to eight years. My residency program (Weill Cornell Medical Center/New York Presbyterian Hospital and Memorial Sloan Kettering Cancer Center) was six years long. Today, neurosurgery residencies are standardized across the country—seven years for all programs. Since 2003, all residency training programs in the United States have restricted work hours for residents to eighty hours per week with at least one day off per seven days. Most programs now have "night float" residents who get to sleep during the day after they have worked all night. Back when I was a resident—in the "days of the giants" as we like to tease current residents—restriction of work hours did not exist. On average, I worked between 100 and 110 hours per week. Some weeks I worked up to 120 hours. Keep in mind, there are only 168 hours in a week! I was on call either every other night or every third night for most of my residency and fellowship. As chief resident, I was on backup call day and night for weeks at a time without any days off, and each night I was awakened multiple times. After being on call, even if I didn't sleep for a minute, I would work the next day. Working weekends and holidays was part of the deal, as neurosurgical emergencies can happen any time.

The first year of my residency training was a general surgery internship. Surgical training programs are very hierarchical, and the intern is at the very bottom of the pecking order. From top to bottom, the order of importance is department chair, other faculty members (also called attending surgeons), chief resident, senior resident, junior resident, and then intern. The intern runs around day and night and does lots of "scutwork," completing mostly basic tasks like checking laboratory results, making sure imaging studies happen, and writing orders. He or she carries a list of all the patients in the hospital being cared for by his or her service (the neurosurgery service, for example). During hospital rounds, the intern writes down tasks to be completed for each patient with open boxes next to them and then checks off these boxes when the tasks are completed. At the end of rounds, the list typically has an overwhelming number of boxes to be checked off. In the meantime, the intern carries a pager—a cell phone these days—that goes off nonstop due to nurses or other doctors trying to reach him or her to write an order, check on a patient who is having a problem, or talk to a patient's family. The intern's reward for doing all this work is getting to go to the operating room to learn how to perform surgeries. With each successive year of residency, the amount of scutwork decreases and the amount of time in the operating room increases.

The internship year is divided into different rotations that typically last one to two months. During my internship, I completed rotations in the burn unit, general surgery, trauma surgery, plastic surgery, cardiac surgery, and neurosurgery. My very first night on call as an intern was on the Fourth of July in the burn unit. I was terrified, as I anticipated tons of patients coming in with burns from fireworks, and I had zero experience treating burn patients. Lots of patients did indeed come in that night, and I got through the night with no disasters—thanks to the burn unit fellow who answered my many questions throughout the night.

The most difficult rotation of my internship by far was a two-month block focused on trauma surgery at Jamaica Hospital in Queens, New York. Jamaica Hospital was essentially the opposite of Jamaica the country (at least for tourists). When tourists go to Jamaica the country, it's for a relaxing beach vacation on a lush tropical island. Working in Jamaica Hospital was like going to hell. The residents on this rotation were divided into two teams. The two teams shared a van for transportation to and from Manhattan. Our team would arrive on a typical weekday at 7:00 A.M.

We then worked all day and all night, usually without sleeping at all, and then saw outpatients in the clinic before driving back, exhausted, at around 3:00 P.M. the following day. The next morning, we would meet around 6:15 A.M. to drive back to the hospital and start all over again. The teams alternated weekends off.

Working weekends at Jamaica Hospital was the most grueling thing I have ever done. It was the surgery equivalent of hell week for Navy SEALs. We would arrive in the van on Saturday morning. We would then work all day and all night for two nights in a row, both Saturday and Sunday. As the intern, I managed up to fifty patients at once, doing my best to care for each patient while my pager went off nonstop. When we had time to eat, we raced down to the cafeteria to scarf down hospital food that was barely edible. To add insult to injury, after forty-eight hours with bad food and little to no sleep, we had to see up to fifty patients in the outpatient clinic before driving back to Manhattan on Monday afternoon. Despite getting the least sleep of any team members, it was the intern's job to drive the van while the more senior residents slept.

I was mostly nonconfrontational as an intern and resident. I understood the pecking order, and I did what I was told. However, I did commit a rare act of defiance after one of these brutal weekends at Jamaica Hospital. I had slept for ten minutes on Saturday night and zero minutes on Sunday night and had worked fifty-six hours in a row. After clinic mercifully ended on Monday afternoon, I could barely see straight, and I knew I was not safe to drive. I handed the keys to the chief resident and said, "I'm sorry, but I'm not driving. I'm going to get us all killed if I do." The chief resident looked at me in shock and disdain, as if I came from another planet. But I didn't give him a choice, so he sat down behind the wheel and drove us home while I slept in the back of the van. I had two simultaneous but conflicting feelings—I felt proud because I had stood up for myself but also ashamed because I was probably the first intern who was too "weak" to drive the van home after the weekend shift.

Like basic training in the military, my two months at Jamaica Hospital were incredibly painful, but they have served me well for the twenty-six years since. To this day, no matter how hard I am working or how exhausted I am, I say to myself, "I can do this. This is nothing compared to Jamaica Hospital." Experiences like these don't exist anymore in residency training in the United States, and many would say that this is a good thing. Long shifts without sleep may result in fatigue-related errors that can harm patients.[1] On the other hand, I am personally grateful to have undergone residency training before the era of work hour restrictions because the intensity made me stronger. Most important, the rigors of residency training taught me to take personal ownership of my patients' outcomes. I am not a shift worker who leaves at the end of my shift no matter what is happening to my patients. I am a doctor whose duty it is to take care of my patients regardless of how sleep-deprived I am or whether or not I am on call. This mentality is lost in some younger members of the medical profession who have grown up in the era of night floats and restricted work hours. Restricting work hours can actually harm patients because many medical errors occur due to inadequate transfer of information during resident handoffs. Some studies have noted increased patient mortality rates during resident handoffs, which are more frequent now than in the era when I trained due to duty hour restrictions.[2] It is hard to know with certainty whether errors from these handoffs are more or less frequent than errors from sleep deprivation would be if there were fewer shift changes. Surgeons argue among themselves about this all the time, and the question has not been well studied.

As an intern or junior resident, it is expected that any assigned tasks will be completed, no matter what. When obstacles are thrown your way, you must find a way to overcome them. If not, you are considered weak. I remember one day when I was tasked with checking a laboratory test that was needed to determine dosing of a "blood thinning" medication. The nurse called me and told me that the patient refused to have his blood drawn for the test. I went to see him and explained the importance of the blood draw. The patient retorted that he was sick of getting stuck with needles and would not give permission for any more blood draws. I called my chief resident and asked him what to do. He replied, with his voice elevated, "God damn it, go back in there and draw that patient's blood!" I went back in the room and tried again to convince the patient, but he would not budge. He said emphatically, "I would rather die than let you draw my blood." Defeated, I called my chief resident and conveyed the patient's words. He replied, "God damn it, Sandberg, go back in that room and do not leave until you have drawn that patient's blood!" I was completely stuck. How can you convince a patient to let you draw his blood when he clearly states that he would rather die? Determined to accomplish my assigned task and not piss off the chief resident further, I returned to the patient's room one final time. I said to him, "Sir, here's the thing. I know you have been clear that you would rather die than let me draw your blood. The problem is that I need to draw your blood to figure out how to dose your medication, and my boss is pretty insistent that I get this done. So, you are welcome to refuse the blood draw, but I am not leaving your room until you say yes. I will stay here all night long if I have to. Neither of us will sleep, and every few minutes I will ask you if you have changed your mind yet." The patient relented, "Fine, you get one stick." He held up a single finger for emphasis. Thankfully, luck was on my side that day, and I got his blood sample with a single needle stick.

During my internship and junior residency years, which included the second and third years of residency, I often carried the service pager during the day and always carried it at night when I was on call. I was the first doctor on our team to be informed by emergency room doctors about a new patient with a neurosurgical emergency or by nurses when an existing patient took a turn for the worse. In emergent situations, I would race to examine the patient, collect pertinent data, and then call the chief resident or attending physician to convey information and propose a plan. I was on the front lines, and I understood the discrepancy between my lack of experience and this huge responsibility. I knew that if my assessment was incorrect, the patient could be seriously harmed or even die. One of the most important lessons I learned from those years was a point emphasized by Dr. Richard Fraser, the former chairman of neurosurgery at Weill Cornell Medical Center. Dr. Fraser would frequently say that "patients eventually always look like their scans." This was a simple statement, but it provided great guidance. He explained that if a patient was wide awake and neurologically normal but his or her CT or MRI scan showed significant bleeding, swelling, or a big stroke, I needed to watch that patient like a hawk because neurological deterioration was imminent. For so many patients with worrisome scans, I did not leave their bedside for hours, and I was there to intervene when their neurological status worsened. On the other hand, if a patient looked terrible but their CT or MRI scan didn't look so bad, they were likely to improve over time. For these patients, I could give their families a glimmer of hope that their loved one had a chance of recovery.

Surgical training includes a gradually escalating level of participation in operations with increasing experience and seniority. For surgical residents, there is sort of an unwritten and unspoken contract between residents and attending surgeons. The residents do all of the "scutwork" for the surgeons, write all the orders, and deal with the daily torture of the pager beeping constantly. By doing so, residents make the attending surgeon's quality of life much better. In return, the attending surgeon teaches the residents to perform operations so they emerge from their long training periods as competent technical surgeons.

I remember being so excited as a junior resident by every new surgical step I was allowed to complete myself in the operating room. At first, I learned to open and close the skin. I was taught by my mentors that nothing less than perfection would be acceptable for every suture that was placed. Like a first kiss, I remember making my first "burr hole," creating a hole in the skull with a high-speed drill. I was nervous that I would plunge the drill through the brain and kill the patient, but a senior resident was there to guide me and make sure I did it safely. I was thrilled the first time I placed a "ventriculostomy," passing a tube through the brain blindly into a fluid space called the lateral ventricle to drain fluid and relieve pressure in an emergency. This was often a lifesaving procedure. I felt the thrilling rush that comes with saving a patient's life with my own hands. I also learned to open and close the dura mater without injuring the brain below.

The first time an attending neurosurgeon allowed me to remove part of a brain tumor under the operating microscope was a monumental experience; I felt like I was on top of the world. Another highlight of every neurosurgery resident's training is clipping an aneurysm for the first time. Aneurysms are outpouchings in blood vessels that can rupture and cause massive bleeding and death. Surgically placing a clip across the neck of an aneurysm prevents the aneurysm from bleeding again. If the surgeon places the clip wrong, the clip could occlude part of a normal blood vessel, causing a stroke, or tear the aneurysm, causing massive bleeding. The first time a resident is entrusted to perform this critical step is a milestone in training because the consequences of making a mistake are so high.

I recall the exhilaration I felt when performing emergent surgeries early in my career. One of the most memorable cases was a baby who was dropped accidentally by his grandfather. The baby became lethargic and was brought to the Emergency Department. A CT scan showed a massive epidural hematoma—just like Garrett's in chapter one—that was shifting the brain over. Without emergency surgery, the baby would likely be dead within hours. We raced to the operating room with the baby and removed the blood clot. The surgery itself was quite easy, and I performed the whole case with supervision from the attending pediatric neurosurgeon. Within hours after surgery, the baby was awake and happily sucking on his bottle. The joy I felt seeing this rapid recovery and the relief of the family was hard to put into words. I felt so honored to have had the opportunity to save this baby's life and share the family's experience of going from the deepest despair to the most profound gratitude. I knew at this moment that choosing to become a neurosurgeon was a great decision for me and that the road ahead would be filled with profoundly meaningful moments.

There were certainly many hard days during residency. I remember one day as a surgical intern during my cardiac surgery rotation. I was assisting in a very stressful and bloody surgery—the repair of a thoracic aortic aneurysm. My job was to retract—to use a metal spatula-like instrument to move structures out of the way so that the attending cardiac surgeon could see and perform the operation. In order to retract correctly, I had to be in a very uncomfortable body position, so I kept shifting my body slightly. When I would do so, the attending cardiac surgeon would yell at me at the top of his lungs to retract better. He probably yelled at me ten times during the operation, and I felt miserable. He never called me by name because he didn't know my name, despite the fact that I had spent the last few weeks taking care of his patients day and night. After the operation was over and things were calm, I went up to him and said, "Sir, I just want to tell you that my name is David Sandberg." I wanted him to know that the person at whom he had just yelled for four hours was a human being with a name. That sentence was all I had to say, and he actually apologized.

On another hard day, I was assisting in neurosurgical cases from early in the morning until the early evening. I was exhausted because I had been up all night on call the night before. The neurosurgeon with whom I was working was in a bad mood the entire day. He barely let me touch an instrument during the operations, and he was mean and condescending. When we finally finished the surgeries, I was mentally and physically depleted. It happened to be my birthday. There would be no birthday dinner or any other celebration that day. I remember feeling down.

But despite all that, in truth, the many highs I experienced as a resident that came from saving people's lives and learning to do increasingly complex procedures completely outweighed any negativity or exhaustion I felt. My good days and moments greatly exceeded the bad ones. I look back on my residency years as some of the best years of my life. I remember one night in 1997 when I was on call. One of my closest friends was in New York City that night for his bachelor party. I couldn't find anyone to trade call days with me, so I couldn't go to the bachelor party. I was really disappointed. It was one of many fun events I would miss during my years of training. The call night was extremely busy. I raced around the hospital seeing consults and doing surgical procedures. Around 3:00 A.M., amid the chaos, I thought to myself that I was probably having more fun than the guys at the bachelor party. I realized both that I must be crazy and that I had definitely chosen the right career.

During their years of training, residents need to decide if they wish to subspecialize within their fields. For me, very early on, I figured out that I wanted to subspecialize in pediatric neurosurgery. I chose this path for many reasons. First, I had an inspiring faculty mentor in pediatric neurosurgery, Dr. Mark Souweidane. Dr. Souweidane is passionate about taking care of kids with neurosurgical problems. He is an immensely talented surgeon and an amazing teacher, and he has an incredible bedside manner. I wanted to be him when I grew up—and still do. I also found myself gravitating toward pediatric cases. I realized that the stakes of challenging surgeries were especially high when the patient was a child, and I thrived on this great responsibility. I loved my days spent on the pediatric wards interacting with children and their families. My research interest, dating from my time as a medical student at Johns Hopkins, was in brain tumors. There was nothing more compelling to me than trying to help find a cure for brain tumors in children. Even on nights when I wasn't on call or expected to be at work, despite my sleep deprivation and lack of time outside the hospital, I would sometimes come in to assist with pediatric neurosurgical cases. Yes, I was a little crazy.

One of the reasons that many residents shy away from pediatric surgical subspecialties is the emotional difficulty that comes with giving bad news to parents about their beloved children. Somehow, early on, I recognized that this was something I was capable of doing. Someone had to be the one to garner the strength to tell a parent that their child had died or would have a horrible outcome. It was a delicate task that had to be done with complete honesty and utter compassion. Certainly, I often had a knot in my throat, and I agonized about these horrible conversations, but it was meaningful to me to have spoken the unspeakable as well as I possibly could. Someone was going to have to give this news to these families, and I felt I could do it as well, if not better, than most because I cared so deeply that it was conveyed with kindness without sacrificing clarity.

After completing residency, I moved to Los Angeles for my pediatric neurosurgery fellowship at Children's Hospital Los Angeles (CHLA). CHLA was an extremely busy center for pediatric neurosurgery, and I trained under two wonderful mentors, Drs. Gordon McComb and Mark Krieger. The fellowship lasted one year, and it was an incredible experience that served as a transition from residency training to independent practice. I had attending privileges and was therefore allowed to do certain cases on my own, but the most difficult cases were supervised by my faculty mentors. I operated and worked day and night. During that year, approximately eight hundred neurosurgical cases were performed on children at CHLA, and I participated in about six hundred of these. There were supposed to be two junior residents on the team—one from the University of Southern California and the other from Dartmouth College. But right before my arrival, I learned that Dartmouth would no longer be sending a resident, and we only had one junior resident for the whole year. This meant that I had to be on call every other night and every other weekend the entire year. It was difficult to take any vacation days because that would leave the junior resident on call two nights in a row, and call nights could be brutal. Moreover, the pediatric neurosurgery service at CHLA simply didn't function without the fellow. That entire year, I only took three working days off—one to attend a family wedding and two to look for housing in Miami where I would be moving after fellowship for my first faculty position. Recognizing my sacrifice, Dr. McComb surprised me at the end of my fellowship by giving me a large bonus that enabled me to buy my first new car.

The last day of my pediatric neurosurgery fellowship was June 30, 2004. This was a huge milestone, the very last day of my neurosurgical training. As of that day, I was a fully trained pediatric neurosurgeon. Since high school, I had completed fifteen years of additional education and training—four years of college, four years of medical school, six years of residency, and one year of fellowship. In fact, this is the fastest path to becoming a pediatric neurosurgeon that exists in the United States. Many pediatric neurosurgeons also do a PhD or participate in extra research years. These individuals may spend up to twenty years after high school before their training is complete. I was one month shy of my thirty-third birthday and possibly the youngest fully trained pediatric neurosurgeon in the country at the time. I was so excited to have my own patients. I felt confident, well trained, and ready for pediatric neurosurgical practice. I also recognized that despite the many years of training, I still had so much to learn.

I was fortunate to learn my trade from some of the most talented neurosurgeons in the world. I appreciated them even more in the years after I completed my training when the tables were turned and I became the teacher rather than the student. It takes great patience to guide a resident through an operation or even a portion of the operation. It is so tempting, at so many moments, to take over and do every part of the operation myself. But I always remember both how hard the residents are working, running around taking care of the patients day and night, and that one day they will need to be out on their own performing operations safely. They cannot learn simply by watching. Of course, my greatest responsibility is to the patient and his or her family, so I frequently take over the critical portion of the case, to the great disappointment of the resident assisting me. Every step of every operation is guided by my knowledge and experience. Some steps can be safely performed by the resident under my watchful eye. Other steps require two sets of hands. And some steps, in my estimation, are best performed by my hands alone. Balancing the dual responsibilities of teaching the next generation of surgeons to be competent and performing the safest operation is a daily challenge for me and for every academic surgeon.

Some parents ask me specifically to promise them that I will be the one doing the operation rather than a trainee. If I make such a promise, I always keep it, but this request puts me in an awkward situation. I take the responsibility of teaching the next generation of neurosurgeons seriously, and I know that if every parent made this request, then the next generation of neurosurgeons would be incompetent. I also remember how I felt as a resident when I was working so hard and my reward was getting to do more and more in the operating room. In reality, portions of most operations require two sets of hands. For example, one surgeon might gently retract a portion of the normal brain with an instrument while the other surgeon biopsies a brain tumor that is thereby exposed. One might think that the trainee would retract and the attending neurosurgeon would perform the biopsy, but there are times when retracting at the perfect angle to expose the tumor is the hard part and taking a biopsy is the easy part. In every case, as the attending neurosurgeon, my greatest responsibility is to the patient and her family, and I personally direct every step of every operation even if my own hands are not performing each maneuver.

After the extensive training neurosurgeons undergo, many of us feel as though we are expected to be able to competently manage any disease within our field. In reality, learning continues throughout our careers and is gained through experience. Many times, fully trained neurosurgery colleagues have asked for my advice about patients or help in the operating room, and I am always flattered. Most commonly, this happens when an adult patient has a condition that is more frequently seen in children. What can be harder to swallow, but is critically important, is to acknowledge when others have expertise I don't have that would benefit my patient. Knowing when to ask for help, even in situations that might be embarrassing, is crucial in order to maximize the possibility of successful patient outcomes.

I recall one such situation vividly. I was five years out of training and feeling confident in my abilities. I was operating on a child who had been in a car accident and had a brain injury that crossed the midline of the brain. These can be dangerous because patients can have catastrophic bleeding during surgery due to injury to the superior sagittal sinus, a huge vein that drains blood from both sides of the brain. And that's exactly what happened. I pulled off fractured pieces of the skull and encountered an explosion of hemorrhage. I needed to repair a laceration in the superior sagittal sinus, but the bleeding was so rapid that I couldn't see exactly where it was coming from. I tried again and again using absorbent cotton sponges to pack off the bleeding. Each time I removed the sponges and tried to repair the superior sagittal sinus, the bleeding erupted again. I tried every trick of the trade to control the bleeding. Nothing worked. In the meantime, the patient required blood transfusion after blood transfusion. After two hours, I was out of ideas.

By chance, a new professor and attending neurosurgeon, Dr. Ross Bullock, had just joined our faculty and happened to be one of the world's experts in neurosurgical trauma. It was midnight, but I swallowed my pride and called Dr. Bullock. It was embarrassing. This was a basic trauma operation, not a delicate aneurysm. I didn't know if he was on call or had the night off, but I needed help. To his credit, Dr. Bullock drove in immediately and joined me in the operating room. By the time he arrived, the bleeding had largely stopped on its own. Now I was really embarrassed that I had asked him to come in, but he handled it graciously. He gave me a few suggestions and went home. I finished the operation, and the patient made a great recovery. Despite the blow to my ego, I knew in my heart that I had done the right thing in asking for help. At the time when I called Dr. Bullock, I thought I could not control the bleeding and that he might have helpful advice. My pride was irrelevant when the life of a child was on the line.

Another time I chose to ask for help was in the case of a toddler who had a benign tumor that was partially solid and partially cystic, fluid filled sac. When these tumors are removed, they normally don't come back for a long time if they come back at all. I operated on this child, and the postoperative MRI showed a complete removal of the tumor. But only a few months later, the cyst associated with the tumor had completely regrown. So, I went back in and removed it again. To my great disappointment, it came back yet again a few months later. I knew I needed to do something different, but I wasn't sure what the best next step was. This was not the kind of tumor that is typically treated with radiation or chemotherapy. It was surgery or nothing, but aggressive surgery had failed twice.

I decided to set my ego aside and get other opinions. I sent the imaging studies to a few colleagues I respect around the country. These colleagues are very senior pediatric neurosurgeons who frequently perform tumor cases. One of them advised against trying to remove the tumor again and instead suggested that I place a catheter in the cyst and attach it to a reservoir through which I could drain the cyst intermittently. This approach worked. We drained fluid from the cyst only a few times, and then the cyst collapsed. Over six years have passed, and no additional intervention has been required for this young boy, who is completely neurologically normal.

These cases showed me the value in swallowing my pride and asking for assistance. There's a feeling that you've done all this training, you've had all this experience, and you shouldn't need help. I'm sure pediatric neurosurgery is not unique in this regard. We are a macho group, whether we are male or female! Asking for help is viewed as a sign of weakness. In fact, as I've learned, the opposite is true. I have observed that the surgeons who feel comfortable asking for help from their colleagues are often those who are the most secure in their knowledge. Surgeons who are more insecure in their knowledge are often reluctant to ask for the input of others, at times to the detriment of their patients. Neurosurgical training does not conclude at the end of residency and fellowship but continues throughout our careers as we learn from our own experiences and from our neurosurgical colleagues. It is incumbent upon us to share our hard-earned knowledge with one another for the benefit of the patients we serve.

3

Hearing the Unthinkable: Helping Families Process a Fatal Diagnosis

I remember vividly on a number of occasions during my childhood when my mother told me that she believes there is no pain worse than the pain parents feel when their child dies. She explained that while the death of any loved one causes heartbreak, mourning the loss of an older relative such as a parent is at least natural and expected. Burying your own child is not part of the natural order of the world, and as a result, it is devastating. As a pediatric neurosurgeon, I have had countless conversations with parents in which I tell them that their child has died or that death or severe disability is imminent or inevitable. When I have these conversations, I always think of my mother's words. I also think about my own children and the despair I would feel if I were on the receiving end of the words I am uttering.

Some conversations stand out in my memory as being particularly brutal. I remember caring for a four-year-old girl who was hit by a car while walking across the street holding her grandmother's hand. The little girl had a horrible traumatic brain injury requiring emergent surgery, with a likely poor prognosis. Her grandmother was instantly killed. Now, it was my job to tell the little girl's mother—who had just received the news that her own mother had died suddenly—that her daughter had a devastating brain injury and could also die. Together with a social worker, I sat down with the little girl's mother and spoke words that were too much for any parent to bear. The little girl underwent emergency surgery and survived, but still suffered permanent neurological impairment from the accident.

It has often struck me that, despite the importance of these conversations, I received no training whatsoever in medical school or residency regarding how to convey bad news to families. For this reason, I always try to take medical students or residents with me when I have tough conversations with families. I tell them that they should observe as many of these conversations as possible with different physicians. They should remember the best of what each physician says, ignore the worst, and develop their own styles.

For me, these conversations boil down to three critical components: compassion, honesty, and listening. I always start by expressing my sorrow. I tell parents that my heart goes out to them, and that I can only imagine how horrible it must be to hear the words that I am saying. I tell them that I have children, and I know how much they love their own child. But I also take a deep breath and tell them the truth. Honesty, while so challenging when the news is unbearable, is critically important in maintaining the trust between the physician and the patient's family. And so, I don't mince words. If a child has died, I don't use phrases that can create confusion like "passed away" or "has gone to a better place." I state clearly, "I am so sorry to tell you this, but your daughter has died." If a child has a severe brain injury with likely permanent neurological impairment, I again don't beat around the bush. I state clearly, "Your son has had a horrible brain injury. Regardless of surgery or other treatments I can offer, he may never walk or talk or eat food on his own or dress himself again. I am so sorry to tell you this devastating news, but I must be completely honest with you." Although words like these are crushing, it is simply unfair to sugarcoat bad news and make things seem better than they are. I have seen so many doctors have wishy-washy conversations in which they never really tell the hard truth, and I have seen how destructive this strategy can be. For example, some parents of children with cancer will continue chemotherapy when there is no realistic possibility of the drugs working. Their children at times experience considerable side effects from these drugs that might not have been administered if the doctor had stated directly that prior patients all had tumor progression on this regimen.

While bad news should be given honestly and directly, doing so without compassion is simply cruel. When giving bad news, I tell parents over and over how sorry I am. I put my arm on their shoulder or hand or offer a hug if it feels appropriate. I listen to them, offering to answer any questions and letting the parents direct the conversation. I spend as much time with them as they need, even sometimes just sitting with them in silence waiting for them to process their thoughts.

I have been asked by family members, friends, and others, "How do you do this? How do you have these conversations?" The answer is that I have these hard conversations because I know that somebody has to do it and because if I were in the shoes of these parents, I know what I would want to hear. When I am delivering bad news to parents, I have no choice but to steel myself, walk into the room, sit down, and have discussions that I know parents will remember forever as among the worst moments of their lives. It's a truly horrible feeling to be the person who shatters a family's world with his words, and I participate in these moments frequently. Even though I have done this countless times, it is never easy.

Over the course of my career, I have seen many different reactions when a parent learns that his or her child has died or receives horrible news that their child has a brain tumor, bleeding in the brain, or another devastating neurological problem. Many parents cry, of course. I have seen some parents literally throw themselves on the floor, wailing uncontrollably and screaming so loud that others are looking from every direction. On some occasions, parents are so emotional that they cannot focus on emergent decisions that need to be made. I have had to say things like, "I cannot imagine what you are going through right now, but I really need your help in deciding whether we should take your son to the operating room right now or not." Some parents stare ahead with no facial expression whatsoever and don't make a sound. Others react with denial or even rage. They simply refuse to believe that what I am saying is true. On a few occasions, parents have simply gotten up and walked away as I am in mid-sentence, as they are unable to hear what has happened to their child. Some parents have a million questions, while others have none. Some parents accept the news immediately, and others simply refuse to accept that nothing can be done to save their child. Upon hearing that surgery will not be offered after traumatic brain injuries, many parents continue to beg over and over for something to be done to save their child regardless of how many times I explain that it's not possible. I teach trainees that each and every one of these reactions is completely normal. There is no normal because as my mother told me, to lose a child is not normal. So we must be prepared for all reactions.

Tragedies involving children can place tremendous stress upon relationships between parents that may have been challenging even before the tragedy. It is incredibly painful to watch parents suffer doubly—both with the cruelty of their child's illness and the strife that this situation creates or exacerbates. In her 1977 book, *The Bereaved Parent*, Harriet Sarnoff Schiff estimated that up to 90 percent of couples who lost a child have serious marital problems within months thereafter and that divorce rates among these couples are higher than in the general population.[1] In a more recent article, noted counselor Reiko Schwab contends that the commonly held belief endorsed by Ms. Sarnoff Schiff that most marriages end in divorce when something devastating happens to a child is not supported by available data.[2] In fact, Schwab argues, many such marriages not only survive, but may ultimately be strengthened.

I certainly have witnessed uncomfortable interactions among parents. Recently, I took care of a young boy who complained of back pain. An MRI scan showed that the cause of his pain was a tumor compressing the spinal cord. When I sat down to go over the results of the MRI scans with his parents and talk about next steps, they were overwhelmed with concerns about surgical risks, subsequent treatments, how to manage their other children, missing work, their son missing school, and a hundred other issues all at once. Pretty quickly, they were at each other's throats. The boy's mother yelled at her husband, "Why are you not crying? You have no empathy! Do you even care?" When the father yelled back, insulting his wife, I intervened, perhaps inappropriately, but I could not help myself. I told them, "I may be overstepping my bounds here, but the horrible news I have given you would put stress on any marriage. Try to treat each other with kindness. Now is the time to take care of each other." I wasn't sure how my words would be received, but they both settled down and neither seemed upset with me.

One of the most devastating conversations I frequently have with parents is conveying that their child has a newly diagnosed malignant brain tumor with a terrible prognosis. The worst of these is Diffuse Intrinsic Pontine Glioma (DIPG), also called Diffuse Midline Glioma. DIPGs are the most dreaded brain tumor that can occur in children. They most commonly are diagnosed in children under age ten. Patients start by having a combination of symptoms such as double vision, unsteady walking, facial weakness, or weakness on one side of the body. This typically leads to an MRI scan that shows a tumor that encompasses and expands much of the brain stem. Removing the tumor surgically is not an option, as the brain stem controls heart rate, blood pressure, and breathing, and the important nerve fibers controlling movement and sensation pass through it. If neurosurgeons tried to remove these tumors surgically, the patients would die. Chemotherapy is completely ineffective against DIPG; no drug, either alone or in combination, has ever been shown to be curative or even to significantly extend survival. Radiation therapy can temporarily alleviate symptoms and extend life expectancy, but only by a few months. And that's all we have to offer besides unproven clinical trials.

Conveying the new diagnosis of DIPG to parents is one of the very hardest conversations I have. I feel like I am delivering one blow after another to the poor parents. First, I must tell them that the symptoms they observed in their child are caused by a brain tumor that was discovered on the MRI. Then I must show them the images and explain why I can't do surgery to remove it. Then, I must essentially destroy all of their hope by telling them that chemotherapy won't work either and that radiation will only help temporarily. Even if radiation therapy prolongs life by a few months, those months are typically miserable as parents see their child lose the ability to swallow food, walk, etc. The average survival after diagnosis is around a year.

Most parents, understandably desperate to save their child, choose radiation therapy and then enroll their child in a clinical trial, hoping that a new treatment will fare better than all the ones that have failed in the past for other children. They hope and pray for a miracle. Rarely, parents will choose no treatment at all. I always counsel parents that there is no wrong decision in these unwinnable circumstances; they must choose the right path for their family and then never look back and feel that they made the wrong decision. If parents want to leave no stone unturned, they should pursue radiation therapy and clinical trials. But if they choose to pursue no treatment at all and go to Disney World or create other special memories in the limited time they have left with their child, this is also not a mistake in my opinion. Sometimes I feel as though we, the doctors, are actually prolonging the process of dying rather than prolonging life when we try to treat these tumors.

Recently, I had one of these agonizing conversations with the parents of Diego, an adorable three-year-old child diagnosed with DIPG. After twenty-four hours of reflection and prayer, the parents decided not to pursue any treatment and to take Diego home to be with his family. I hugged his mom and dad and told them that they were wonderful parents and again expressed my sorrow. And yet again, as I have done so many times during my years as a pediatric neurosurgeon, I went home and hugged my own kids a little longer than I had the day before.

Some malignant brain tumors that occur in children have better outcomes than DIPG, but many children ultimately do not survive despite intensive treatments. Two such tumors are medulloblastoma and ependymoma, both of which are a primary focus of my own research. Both are rare tumors that affect children more frequently than adults and can sometimes be cured by surgery and other treatments. However, when these tumors recur after initial treatments, additional interventions are rarely curative, and parents must make impossible decisions over and over again. How long should they keep fighting, and at what cost? Should they agree to a second surgery when the tumor grows back months or years after the first surgery, knowing that it will likely buy their child more time but also risk hurting him or her neurologically? How about a third surgery, or a fourth, fifth, or sixth? Should they try yet another chemotherapy agent despite the fact that all of the others failed, and some cause serious side effects?

In these impossible situations, I view my role as that of a counselor and hopefully a friend. I relay the hard facts—as gently as I can but with complete honesty—and I spend a lot of time listening and figuring out where the parents are emotionally. I answer their questions about all options. Perhaps the best question, which people often ask, is, "What would you do if this were your own child?" I always answer this question directly, and the answer varies depending upon the situation. Some parents are surprised when I say that I would choose no further treatment for my child. Others are equally surprised when I convey, in different situations, that while the odds are against us, I would personally continue to fight and would choose yet another surgery or other treatment. My recommendations when asked this question are based upon a blend of science—an understanding of the disease process and statistical likelihood of survival or recovery—and intuition. The intuition component includes factors such as my personal experiences with similar patients in the past, the amount of suffering that would accompany the surgery or treatment, and my assessment of the mental state of the child and the child's parents.

I chose to become a pediatric neurosurgeon for many reasons, one of which was the awe I have for the deep resilience of children and their parents. The majority of kids I treat have great outcomes, and one of the most rewarding aspects of my job is giving great news to parents after a successful operation. The overwhelming gratitude I receive, including hugs and tears of joy, provides me with satisfaction that is hard to quantify. These conversations come easily and increase my eagerness to come back to work the next day, even though I have been doing this job for many years. I have realized over the years that the hard conversations, in which I deliver bad news, are not only critically important but can be rewarding in their own way. When having the devastating conversations I described in this chapter, I pride myself on doing the best possible job that I can in providing both loving compassion and brutal honesty. Most of the time, even when sharing horrible news, I am able to feel a connection with parents and can sense their gratitude for the manner in which I have spoken the unspeakable. Parents can be so hard on themselves when their child has a fatal condition, and I am always hopeful that I have helped parents make impossible choices without their second-guessing their decisions and beating themselves up unfairly. After the toughest conversations, I go home and count my own blessings, and I hope that the next day is one where I deliver only good news to families.

4

The Greatest Reward: Saving the Life of a Child

I t was over twenty years ago, but I remember the moment I met Marcela as if it were yesterday. Marcela was an eight-year-old girl who looked younger than her age. She was thin and frail but adorable. Marcela's mother was at her bedside and looked very worried. They were surrounded by many other extremely sick children in the crowded pediatric wards of Hospital Escuela, the public teaching hospital in Tegucigalpa, Honduras. Many of these children were destined to die, and the most tragic thing was that so many of them had curable conditions. It was a heartbreaking scene that I carry with me to this day. I wished I could provide every one of these kids with the care that was available in my own country. For some reason, among all of these beautiful children, Marcela captured my heart. I knew that I had to find a way to help this child.

When I met Marcela, I was a neurosurgery resident in my fourth year of training. Because of my interest in pediatric neurosurgery in developing countries, I was spending my four weeks of vacation volunteering at the Hospital Escuela. Hospital Escuela serves the 90 percent of the population of Honduras's capital that cannot afford care in private hospitals. The hospital was filthy and overcrowded. The pediatric ward overflowed with children suffering or dying. Many of them had huge brain tumors or other problems that would have been treated months or even years earlier if they had lived in a more developed country or if their family had the means to pay for private care. Hospital Escuela did not have the staff or capability to properly care for them, and many died before ever receiving operations that could have easily saved their lives.

I met Marcela in the back corner of the pediatric ward, and I learned her history from her mother, Aracely. Marcela was a previously healthy girl who attended a public school in Tegucigalpa that had a special program for children talented in music. For about two years, she had insatiable thirst and was constantly drinking water and then urinating frequently. The cause of her thirst and frequent urination was not diagnosed by her pediatrician despite multiple visits to the office. In December 2000, she began to have decreased appetite. In April 2001, she began to have daily headaches and intermittent vomiting.

Because of the vomiting, she was referred to a gastro-enterologist who performed an endoscopy, which found no abnormalities in her upper GI tract. In early May 2001, Marcela began to complain of altered vision. An ophthalmologist determined that Marcela had bitemporal hemianopsia—she could see objects in a narrow field right in front of her but could not see in the periphery. Finally, over two years after her initial symptoms, a CT scan of her brain was performed that showed a massive brain tumor. The tumor was causing Marcela's visual problems by compressing the optic chiasm, a structure in the brain which carries fibers from both optic nerves. Her thirst and frequent urination were caused by the tumor's effects on the pituitary gland, a condition called diabetes insipidus.

Marcela's case was extreme in terms of how long after her symptoms the tumor was diagnosed, but a delay in the diagnosis of a brain tumor in a child in the developing world did not surprise me. Even in the United States, such delays are often the rule rather than the exception. Pediatricians evaluate so many children daily who have headaches, vomiting, or other symptoms that are usually caused by common problems such as viral illnesses. The average pediatrician may see only one child with a brain tumor in his or her entire career. Our health care system is not equipped to send every child with a head-ache or vomiting for imaging studies of the brain, as the overwhelming majority of these studies would reveal no abnormality. Pediatricians often feel incredible guilt when the diagnosis of a brain tumor has been delayed. I feel great sympathy for these pediatricians because it is no easy task to determine which of the one hundred kids they saw with vomiting in any given month needs a scan. In the overwhelming majority of cases that I have seen in my career, the pediatrician was not at fault. I have had long conversations with pediatricians reassuring them that their care was completely appropriate.

Parents additionally often feel incredible guilt when the diagnosis of a brain tumor is made months after initial symptoms were noted. Many mothers and fathers are convinced that both the problem and its delay in being discovered are their fault. "It must have been something I did during pregnancy." "It must have been the food I fed her." "It must have been something he was exposed to in our home or neighborhood." "I should have taken her to the doctor sooner." "I should have taken her to a different doctor when her pediatrician said it was a virus." I have heard each of these statements and others like them countless times, and I often tell crying parents over and over again that none of this is their fault. They usually keep crying so I say it over and over. "This is not your fault." So many times, no matter what I say, parents don't believe it, and they carry an unfair burden of guilt. This guilt, in addition to the devastation parents already feel because their child has a brain tumor, can be overwhelming. Many parents simply cannot accept that there is nobody to blame and that even if there were, it would not help anyway.

Marcela's family consulted with a private neurosurgeon in Tegucigalpa who advised a craniotomy, a big operation to take off a piece of the skull and remove the tumor, which he believed to be a craniopharyngioma, a type of tumor that is typically initially treated with surgery. Marcela's parents could not afford this neurosurgeon's surgical fee, so they took her to Hospital Escuela, the public hospital, and this is where I first met her. When I saw Marcela's imaging studies of the brain, I knew immediately that her tumor was not a craniopharyngioma. It had the classic appearance of another type of tumor called a germinoma, for which the appropriate treatment was *not* surgical resection. In the United States, this tumor would be treated with radiation therapy, and sometimes additionally with chemotherapy, with a 90 percent cure rate.

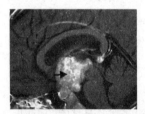

Figure 3. *Marcela's MRI showing massive brain tumor with imaging features typical of germinoma. The arrow sits in the center of the tumor.*

At this point, I was stuck. I knew what needed to be done for this child, but I had no way of making it happen. I was only a resident, not a fully trained neurosurgeon, and I was scheduled to leave Honduras in just over a week. When I had a free moment later that day, I went to a pay phone outside the hospital. I called Dr. Souweidane, my pediatric neurosurgery faculty mentor in New York. When I told Dr. Souweidane about Marcela, his response was immediate and definitive—we have to find a way to bring this child to New York! When I heard these words, I was filled with a sudden burst of hope. That hope quickly faded when I started thinking about all of the logistical barriers in our way: Would we be able to get travel visas for Marcela and her mother to enter the United States? Would she be safe to travel on an airplane? Where would she and her mom stay in New York? Who would feed them and take care of them? Could funds be raised to pay for expensive treatments in New York? How would we handle follow-up care in Honduras? I was overwhelmed by these details.

Dr. Souweidane and I both got to work immediately. I prepared letters for Marcela's parents to take to the United States Embassy requesting travel visas for Marcela and her mother—explaining that this trip would save Marcela's life. I helped her get an appointment quickly at the U.S. Embassy, which was not an easy feat. Dr. Souweidane convinced the administrators of our hospital (New York Presbyterian Hospital/Weill Cornell Medical Center) to allow us to bring Marcela for treatment as a charity case. He also found a local organization in New York that offered to take care of travel expenses, housing, and food for Marcela and her mother. In the meantime, it was time for me to leave Honduras and go back to New York to resume my residency training. One of the last things I did before leaving was to go out to breakfast with Marcela's parents, Aracely and Juan Carlos. They had limited means, but they generously insisted on treating me to breakfast. At that meal, I promised that I would not forget Marcela and that I would do everything in my power to bring her to New York, but I warned them that I might not be able to make it happen. They gave me a photo of Marcela that I put in my wallet, and it stayed there for many years thereafter. When we said goodbye, I had no idea whether I would ever see them or their daughter again.

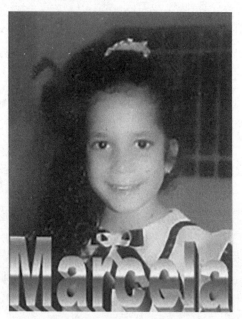

Figure 4. *Marcela's photo from 2001 that stayed in my wallet for years.*

By the end of May 2001, Marcela had been discharged from Hospital Escuela and I was back in New York. Her parents and I anxiously awaited approval from both the U.S. Embassy and our hospital in New York, both of which we miraculously received! I was joyous and hopeful as we purchased plane tickets and prepared for Marcela's arrival in New York.

But we were not out of the woods. Just days before her planned trip, on June 9, 2001, Marcela's headaches became more intense and she started vomiting repeatedly. Her parents took her back to Hospital Escuela, where a CT scan showed that the tumor had caused worsened hydrocephalus—a blockage of the normal pathways whereby cerebrospinal fluid (CSF) produced in the brain circulates resulting in high pressure in the brain. Dr. Tulio Murillo, an outstanding neurosurgery resident at Hospital Escuela, placed a ventriculoperitoneal shunt in the middle of the night. This was a lifesaving operation to divert fluid from Marcela's brain to her abdomen, and Marcela immediately felt better. Several days later, she was discharged from Hospital Escuela, and she and her mother boarded a plane to New York.

The next challenge that arose—the day before Marcela's planned arrival—was that we had no place for Marcela and her mother to stay once they arrived in New York. The local organization that purchased their plane tickets had also promised to arrange housing, but this fell through. I asked my girlfriend, Amy Schefler, who was a medical student at Cornell, to let me temporarily move into her small studio apartment, and I prepared my own studio apartment for Marcela and her mother. Amy and I went together to the airport to pick up Marcela and her mom. We nervously awaited their arrival, counting the hours until the flight landed. When they arrived, it was late at night, and Marcela looked lethargic and unwell, with her mother carrying her in her arms like a baby. I worried to myself that we might have gotten her to New York too late—and tried to keep smiling at them to make sure they could not see this concern on my face.

We brought Marcela and her mother back to my apartment. The next morning, we admitted Marcela to the hospital. We performed a new CT scan, which showed that the shunt placed by Dr. Murillo was adequately draining one side of the brain, but the fluid space (called the lateral ventricle) on the other side of the brain was still very enlarged. On June 13, 2001, Dr. Souweidane and I performed a minimally invasive endoscopic surgical procedure that accomplished three goals: (1) we biopsied the tumor to confirm the diagnosis; (2) we performed a septostomy—making an opening in a structure called the septum pellucidum to enable the shunt placed by Dr. Murillo to drain fluid from both sides of the brain; and (3) we sampled the CSF in the brain to send for various tests that would also confirm the diagnosis. The diagnosis of germinoma was confirmed, and Marcela went on to receive radiation therapy across the street at

Memorial Sloan Kettering Cancer Center. The tumor melted away with radiation therapy, and it never recurred. Over the next few months, her vision improved back to normal and her appetite recovered. I arranged charitable donations of medicines needed to treat hormone deficiencies caused by the tumor. Three months after her arrival, Marcela and her mother were back on a plane home to Honduras for a reunion with her father, brother, sister, and many other family members marked by many hugs and tears of joy.

Over the years that followed, I kept in close touch with Marcela and her family. She continued to thrive, was a straight A student, and had no medical problems other than the hormone issues that were controlled by the medicines I shipped to her. The next time I saw Marcela in person was three years later. Amy and I had become very close to Marcela and her family, and we brought them to New York for our wedding as a wedding gift to ourselves. Marcela and her younger sister, Katherine, were the flower girls at our wedding. I will never forget watching them walk down the aisle and seeing the reaction of our wedding guests. There was not a dry eye in the entire room.

Fast-forward twenty-one years—Marcela is now a medical student in Costa Rica, where she has moved with her family to escape violence in Honduras. She plans to become a pediatrician. She is a warm and compassionate young woman, and her own experiences as a patient will make her an extraordinary doctor in the coming years.

Marcela's story is a remarkable one. The fact that she is alive today defied the odds in so many ways. She had the good fortune to be admitted to Hospital Escuela during my visit, and so many pieces fell into place that could have easily not worked out. It took an extraordinary amount of work both by me and by Dr. Souweidane to enable her to receive lifesaving treatment in New York. For me, the experience of caring for Marcela during my residency training and beyond was a formative one that taught me many lessons.

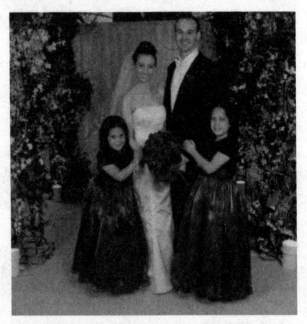

Figure 5. *Marcela (right) and Katherine, the flower girls at our wedding in 2003.*

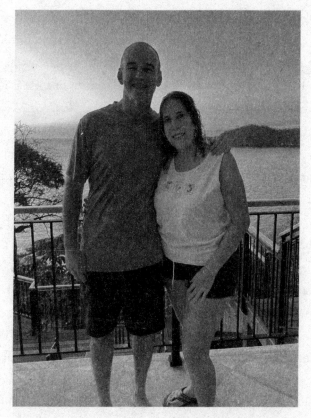

Figure 6. *A recent (2022) picture of Marcela and me from a family vacation in Costa Rica.*

First, I learned something that I understood even more profoundly years later when I had my own kids: that the value of a single human life—especially that of a child—is immeasurable. I witnessed the despair of Marcela's mother in Honduras as she watched her precious daughter suffer from a life-threatening illness. I then witnessed Aracely's joy as Marcela recovered physically and when I showed her that the tumor was gone on a follow-up MRI after radiation. I better appreciated a saying from the Talmud—a sacred Jewish text—that my parents had taught me growing up: "A person who saves one life is as if he saved a whole world."[1] I understood that, for Marcela's family, Dr. Souweidane and I had saved their entire world. As a physician, the satisfaction this gave me, and that I have thankfully experienced many times since, is too profound to put into words.

Sadly, I learned firsthand how unfair the world is. By sheer chance alone, my own children were born in the United States to parents with the means to care for all of their needs. If, God forbid, my own daughter had a life-threatening illness, she would receive the very best care available. We were able to provide this for Marcela, but not for so many other children with curable illnesses that I met at the Hospital Escuela or on subsequent trips abroad. Because it is impossible financially and logistically to bring every sick child from a low- or middle-income country to a developed country for care, I feel compelled to help in any way I can to improve the care that can be delivered locally. I will expand on this in chapter 9.

And finally, I learned from my experience taking care of Marcela how much we gain as individuals by going out of our way to help others, sometimes in unexpected ways. I am certain—and I say this with sincerity—that Marcela and her family did just as much for me as I did for them. As I described earlier, when Marcela and her mother were about to leave for New York, their housing fell through at the last minute, and they wound up staying in my apartment for three months. The only thing I asked of my girlfriend, Amy, other than sharing her apartment, was to make a welcome sign for us to bring to the airport since Amy is a better artist than I am. Amy didn't speak a word of Spanish, and Marcela and her mother did not speak a word of English. Yet, over the next three months, Amy astonished me. Night after night, I would finish my work as a resident late in the evening and then go to my apartment to check on Marcela and her mom. Despite the fact that Amy was a busy medical student, every night I would find her sitting on the floor playing with Marcela. Amy began to learn Spanish from Marcela and her mom, and the love that she displayed to this little girl made me realize that Amy had to be the mother of my own children one day. There is no doubt in my mind that Amy's interactions with Marcela were the final step in convincing me that I was meant to marry Amy—and I am truly lucky that I must have done something to convince her that she wanted to marry me, too! Amy and I have been happily married for over twenty years and have two children of our own.

As I look back on my years spent as a pediatric neurosurgeon, it is hard to adequately express the joy that I have felt when given the opportunity to save the lives of many children. Each of these children is a treasure whose value is immeasurable to his or her parents, grandparents, siblings, and other loved ones. The gratitude that I receive from these families makes any negative aspects of my chosen path—exhausting hours, frustrating encounters with insurance companies, burdensome documentation in medical records, etc.—simply melt away. I receive many gifts from families, which often make me a little embarrassed. I tell parents that I don't need gifts, as my greatest gift is the opportunity to take care of their children. What does mean the world to me are the notes that accompany these gifts, so many of which are filled with the most beautiful and touching words. I save these notes, and one day, probably at the end of my career, I will pull them all out and read them again with great pride.

One thing that I must say is that I personally receive too much credit for saving the life of each individual child. I am often the most visible face of a team that includes many people who pour their hearts and souls into caring for each of our patients. Our medical assistants and clinic nurses go above and beyond for every patient and their family and go out of their way to show parents that they sympathize with the anxieties that accompany having a sick child. Neurosurgery residents and physician assistants run around the hospital taking care of patients and enable emergency care to proceed expeditiously. Hospital nurses and child life specialists shower each child with kindness and love. Anesthesiologists keep children safe and comfortable during surgery, overcoming unexpected challenges that can arise in any operation. Custodial staff race to clean operating rooms before surgical emergencies, working as fast as they can knowing the situation at hand. Many times, I personally receive all of the praise that really should be shared with so many others. And so, I want to encourage families to spread the wealth when it comes to gifts and notes to others besides their child's surgeon. These individuals do not do what they do in order to receive recognition, but expressions of gratitude mean the world to all of us.

5

Coping with Complications: When the Patient Is Worse after Surgery

I will never forget seeing James walk into my office. The reason I will never forget this is that after the surgery I performed, James never walked again for the rest of his life. This is an undeniable fact, and it is something that I have had to live with ever since.

James was a very polite and likeable fifteen-year-old boy who came into my clinic together with his father. James's father's face was drawn tight, and he had wrinkles under his eyes. James had been complaining of back pain for a number of weeks, and his pain was worsening by the day. His father had taken him to his primary doctor for the pain, but nothing much had been done and imaging of the spine was not performed. James then developed weakness in his legs, and he was embarrassed to share that he was now having urinary accidents because he could no longer control his bladder. James walked into my office hunched over, grimacing from the pain, and limping due to leg weakness. He could barely walk without assistance, but he walked in on his own two feet. When an MRI scan was performed, it showed the problem clearly—a large tumor within the spinal cord in the thoracic region (in the middle of his back).

When I examined James in the office, his neurological examination corresponded perfectly to the tumor visualized on the MRI scan. The strength and sensation in his arms were normal. This was expected, as upper extremity strength and sensation are controlled by the cervical spinal cord in the neck. Motor and sensory fibers from the brain travel down to the cervical spinal cord, and nerve roots that come from the spinal cord in this region allow the arms and hands to function. On the other hand, lower extremity function and bowel/bladder function are controlled by nerve roots which arise from the lumbar spinal cord in the lower part of the back. Any condition injuring the spinal cord above this level—such as James's tumor in the thoracic region—can damage nerve fibers within the spinal cord intended to reach the legs and also the sacral nerve roots that control bowel and bladder function. So, it was no surprise when I examined James that his legs were weak and that when I touched his body to assess his sensation,

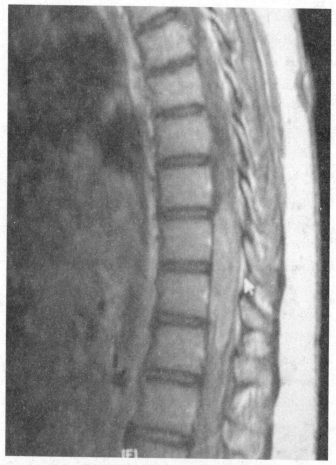

Figure 7. *MRI scan showing James's large tumor, marked by arrow, expanding the spinal cord.*

he could barely feel anything below the waist. It was also logical that he was having urinary accidents.

In the office, I showed James and his father the MRI scan, and I explained why he was having severe back pain, weakness, and problems controlling urination. I told them that we needed to perform surgery to diagnose what type of tumor he had, as the specific pathologic diagnosis—made by a pathologist looking at tumor tissue under a microscope—would determine which treatments would follow. Additionally, I would try to remove as much tumor as I could safely. I went over the risks of surgery, including worsening of his existing problems, but I assured James and his father that I would do everything I could to avoid this worsening. We admitted James to the hospital and planned for surgery the next day.

Before starting the operation, after James had been put to sleep, I had a technician place small electrodes in various muscles in James's legs in order to monitor Motor Evoked Potentials (MEPs) and Somatosensory Evoked Potentials (SSEPs) during surgery. MEPs assess whether the spinal cord can send impulses to specific muscles that enable leg movement; SSEPs assess whether the spinal cord's pathways that enable sensation are intact. MEPs and SSEPs make surgery safer by allowing us to detect disruptions in the function of the spinal cord in real time.

After the electrodes were placed and James was positioned and prepped, I made an incision in James's back with a scalpel. After dissecting through the muscles on top of the spine, I cut the bones overlying the spinal cord with a high-speed drill. Under the bones was the dura mater, the tough membrane that covers the spinal cord (in addition to the brain). I localized the tumor with an intraoperative ultrasound machine and brought in a high-powered operating microscope. As I used my knife to open the dura, it was immediately clear that the spinal cord was very swollen. I quickly opened the rest of the exposed dura—which extended both above and below the tumor—to create room for the spinal cord.

As I made a small opening in the surface of the spinal cord, the tumor started squeezing out like toothpaste under pressure. I suctioned out some obvious tumor to relieve the pressure. As I did so, the technician monitoring James's spinal cord function with the electrodes called out to me that there was a sudden decrease in both MEPs and SSEPs. This meant that the motor and sensory function in James's legs were potentially in jeopardy. I made sure that James's blood pressure and other vital signs were normal—even as my own blood pressure was shooting through the roof—and that there was no obvious problem in the surgical field. Within less than a minute, I was informed that all motor and sensory function in his lower extremities was gone, and I knew that we were in big trouble. Losing these signals completely was a worrisome sign—a neurosurgeon's nightmare. Barring a technical problem with the monitoring, I knew that this poor kid may never move his legs again. And that is exactly what happened.

In the meantime, I sent a piece of the tumor that I had removed to the pathologist. Because of the absent MEPs and SSEPs, I didn't remove any additional tumor. I waited impatiently for the pathologist to call back into the room. It was only about fifteen minutes later but it felt like forever. Finally, the pathologist called into the room with the worst news—the diagnosis was glioblastoma multiforme, a malignant tumor with a very poor prognosis that occurs more often in the brain but can also occur in the spinal cord. With this diagnosis, there would be no benefit to removing more tumor, and the spinal cord was less swollen after opening the dura and removing the obvious tumor that had presented to the surface when I opened the spinal cord. So, I closed by suturing in a graft of a dural substitute to give extra space for the spinal cord in case there was worsened swelling postoperatively. I then sutured closed the spine muscles and skin.

After I finished the operation, I waited anxiously in the operating room for James to wake up. As he woke up, he moved his arms perfectly but could not move his legs at all. My heart sank.

My next task was to go out to the waiting room and give two horrible pieces of news to James's father. First, I had to tell him that his son had a cancer of the spinal cord for which there was no cure. As if that wasn't devastating enough, I also had to tell James's dad that his son had lost the ability to move his legs and that this ability may never come back. I took a deep breath and tried to summon up inner strength. I went out to the waiting room and led James's dad to a private room. The words that came out of my mouth were painfully difficult for me to speak but completely unbearable for a parent to hear.

The events that occurred in James's case were unusual and had never happened before in the many patients with spinal cord tumors upon whom I had previously operated. I had never seen complete loss of all motor and sensory function after making a small opening in the spinal cord and removing obvious tumor while protecting the normal spinal cord. In retrospect, after considerable reflection on every step of the operation, I could not think of anything that I could have done differently that would have changed the outcome. But any change in neurological function after a surgery that makes the patient worse than he or she was beforehand is, appropriately, considered a complication. It was my surgical complication, and I knew that.

Extreme situations like this are, thankfully, very rare. Most pediatric neurosurgical procedures have positive outcomes. However, complications occur more commonly than we would like to admit. In one review from the Netherlands, complications recognized during the operation occurred in 3.5 percent of pediatric neurosurgery procedures.[1] In another article reviewing rates of complications at the Hospital for Sick Children in Toronto—one of the most outstanding pediatric neurosurgery centers in the world—complications (both intraoperative and postoperative) occurred in 16.4 percent of pediatric neurosurgery procedures.[2]

When a major complication occurs, there are so many things going through my mind at once. In the midst of a crisis, the first thing I am thinking (along with "Oh, shit!") is whether there is anything I can do to reverse the problem. Once the heat of the moment has passed—for example, as I waited for James to wake up—I am praying that things aren't as bad as they seem. When I am forced to confront the reality that the situation is indeed horrible, more thoughts race through my mind. First and foremost, I reflect on whether I could have done anything differently to prevent the problem. I feel sadness for the child and his or her parents. I feel anxiety about explaining the situation to the child's parents. I feel additional worry about presenting the case in Morbidity and Mortality conference (more on this in a moment). I am resolved to be one hundred percent truthful with the parents, to take ownership of the situation, and to be compassionate.

Over the years, I have seen surgeons handle complications in many different ways. One extreme approach I have seen is that some surgeons refuse to even consider the possibility that they could have done something better. I could say to myself, "I am an experienced surgeon, and I trained at the very best places. I did my best, and that's all I can do. This could happen to any surgeon, and it's not my fault." My honest opinion is that surgeons who approach complications in this manner are not worthy of the great honor of taking care of patients. On the other extreme, some surgeons are so devastated by surgical complications that they struggle to be effective for future patients. They succumb to self-doubt and shy away from difficult operations, sometimes to the detriment of their patients. It has been my observation over the years that a large number of surgeons fall into both of these categories.

I believe that the best way for a surgeon to approach surgical complications is in a balanced way that steers clear of each of these two extremes. Honest and deep reflection on the case is imperative in order to learn any possible lessons that could potentially prevent the same complication from occurring in the future. I have lost many hours of sleep after complications. I lie awake hour after hour thinking about what went wrong and whether I should have done anything differently. I review every detail about the case, starting with my initial encounter with the patient and their family and ending with the present moment. I ask myself hard questions—and I demand honest answers from myself. Was the surgery definitely indicated? Were there alternatives I should have considered? Is there anything I could have done better in my preoperative discussion with the family? In my discussion of risks and benefits associated with the surgery, did I adequately discuss the specific complication that occurred?

Every surgery has risks and benefits, and surgery should only be offered if the risks outweigh the benefits. Honest preoperative discussions about surgery must convey the risks and benefits associated with the procedure as well as alternative options to surgery. These discussions are extremely important, and tensions are often high, especially when the patient is a child. As a father, I can only imagine the anxiety parents feel when hearing that their child needs brain or spine surgery. Parents want reassurance that their child is going to be okay, that their nightmare is going to have a happy ending. Some surgeons, usually with good intentions, downplay the risks in order to help parents cope with their anxiety. While doing so may make families feel more comfortable preoperatively, parents may feel justifiably angry if a complication occurs that they were not warned about preoperatively. Other surgeons, trying to avoid this situation, go over every complication they can possibly imagine in great detail, leaving patients and their families terrified.

I remember hearing from one of my mentors that if you are getting consent from a parent for a neurosurgical procedure and the parent is not crying, you probably have not obtained a truly informed consent. While I would never want to make someone cry on purpose, there is truth to this statement. During preoperative discussions, I am direct about the risks of the operation while explaining why the benefits still outweigh the risks. I also try to reassure parents by describing successful outcomes in similar previous cases and by promising to do everything in my power to minimize the possibility of complications.

I often tell frightened parents, "I have to tell you all of these horrible things that could happen, but I genuinely think that this will have a happy ending." There are occasions, however, when complications occur that are so rare or so unexpected that it does not occur to me to mention them preoperatively. These occasions require considerable discussion with families regarding why the specific complication that occurred was not discussed preoperatively. These conversations can be especially difficult as parents are sometimes angry that I did not warn them of the specific complication that happened in their child's case.

For surgeries that are especially risky, such as large tumors deep within the brain, I have found that some families are so traumatized when the risks are explained to them that they have a hard time processing the information. So many times, after I have gone over in great detail some pretty scary things that can happen (such as serious bleeding or new weakness or inability to talk or walk), a parent will ask, "But my child will be okay, right?" Part of me wants to respond, "Huh? Did you not hear what I just said?" Of course, I would never do so because I understand that the parent is terrified and just needs reassurance. I am stuck between two bad choices: leaving the parent traumatized or providing false reassurance by promising that nothing bad will happen. My approach is to respond by saying something like, "The risks I described are real, but I promise to do everything in my power to return your baby to you without any of these bad things happening."

The reactions that patients and families have after a complication occurs vary widely. Some accept the explanation of the physician and focus exclusively on the recovery of their loved one. Some are so empathetic that they actually feel bad for the surgeon and ask, "Are you okay?" Others feel anger, and some direct this anger at the surgeon. Dr. Meinhard Bienst, a neurosurgeon from Honduras who is a close friend of mine once told me, only half-joking, "When my surgeries go great, my patients say, 'Thank God!' God gets the credit for the surgery going well, not me. But when a complication occurs, they always blame me, not God." While I laughed when Meinhard said this, my own experience is that when surgeries go well the majority of patients are actually incredibly grateful and give the surgeon plenty of credit. I am frequently showered with praise, sometimes so much so that I feel embarrassed.

After a complication occurs, I reflect in depth about technical aspects of the surgery, postoperative care, and postoperative communication with the family. I review the preoperative imaging studies again to see if clues can be found that could have predicted the occurrence of the complication. I think about the surgical approach I chose and whether there were equal or better alternatives. I replay every step of the operation in my mind and assess whether any technical error occurred. I additionally consider whether the postoperative care was optimal and whether everything possible was done to mitigate the effects of the complication. And finally, I evaluate the effectiveness of my communication with the patient and his or her family after the complication was recognized.

And then there's the Morbidity and Mortality conference, M&M. At this conference, held frequently at academic medical centers, attendees discuss surgical complications to make sure the care provided meets accepted standards. This is an extremely important process that is educational for all attendees. But, boy, it is painful for the surgeon who had the complication! Imagine your worst or most embarrassing day. Now, imagine having every detail of that day, with pictures, shown on a large screen to everyone you work with, including your boss, your colleagues, doctors in training, students, and people you have never seen before. The night before a complication of mine is presented at M&M conference is rarely a good night's sleep for me. Despite the angst I feel, I am a huge supporter of this process. I learn something almost every time my own complications are presented, and I learn from the complications of my colleagues as well. I am certain that the lessons learned at these conferences lead to better outcomes for future patients of surgeons who are humble enough to learn from their mistakes. Attending hundreds of these conferences over the years has made me a better surgeon.

In some situations, as in James's case, the process of honest self-reflection and presentation in the M&M conference does not lead to a "smoking gun" regarding what should be done better in future operations. James's complication was probably the unavoidable consequence of a horrible disease. Sadly, he passed away eleven months later from his aggressive cancer, unrelated to the surgery. In other cases, thankfully rare in my own career, a complication can be attributed to a mistake that the surgeon made. There are mistakes in judgment such as not offering a surgery that should have been offered or offering the surgery too late. There are surgeries that should never have been considered in the first place because the benefits did not outweigh the risks. And then—the hardest pill for a surgeon to swallow—there are technical errors made during the surgery. Every neurosurgeon I know has made technical errors in his or her career, and they are awful for the surgeon's psyche. All complications are stressful, but potentially preventable technical errors weigh heaviest on the surgeon's mind. This is because the surgeon's self-esteem is highly bound up in the notion that our steady hands can work near the most important structures without causing harm. Technical errors are a huge blow to our egos.

In some states more than others, doctors must additionally worry about medical malpractice lawsuits. Thankfully, such suits are relatively rare in Texas where I practice, so I seldom focus on this. However, when I lived in New York, California, and Florida—all states where the medicolegal climate is more heated—I thought about lawsuits much more frequently. According to a recent study, approximately 20 percent of all neurosurgeons in the United States are named as defendants in a malpractice lawsuit each year, and nearly all neurosurgeons are named as defendants at some point in their careers.[3] Neurosurgeons are sued more frequently than any other medical specialist.[4] The medicolegal landscape in the U.S. is very complex and multilayered. It protects patients and families and holds physicians to a very high standard, which has helped produce the highest level of medical excellence in our country. On the other hand, it also produces a tremendous amount of stress for doctors and for patients, and results in countless unindicated medical tests and procedures.

This brings me to one of the most painful situations I have dealt with in my career—a case in which I was a defendant in a lawsuit. Although almost every neurosurgeon I know has been named in a lawsuit—some many times—I never thought it would happen to me. I knew that I would never actually commit malpractice by doing something that was below established standards of care like not coming to the hospital in the middle of the night to handle an emergency or performing an unneccessary surgery. I knew that if I had a surgical complication or a bad outcome I would focus intently on honest and compassionate communication with the patient and his or her family. I naively assumed that I would thereby avoid being sued. I was wrong.

The patient was Sara, a young girl who was under my care during my fellowship at Children's Hospital Los Angeles. Sara had been born severely premature, at twenty-six weeks gestational age. Her long stay in the neonatal intensive care unit had been complicated by spontaneous bleeding in the brain that eventually led to hydrocephalus—increased pressure in the brain caused by her brain's lack of ability to properly circulate the fluid it produced. Her hydrocephalus had been treated with a shunt—a catheter that drains fluid from the brain to the abdomen with an intervening valve that regulates the amount of fluid drained.

Now four years old, Sara was an inpatient at another hospital in Los Angeles. She had been brought to the Emergency Department by her mother for severe abdominal pain. As it turned out, she had appendicitis, but there was a delay in diagnosing this by the doctors treating her. By the time her appendicitis was recognized, the appendix had ruptured, and pus had spread throughout her abdominal cavity. Appendicitis is most commonly treated with a simple operation, but in this case, the pediatric surgeon at the outside hospital recommended antibiotics only rather than surgery. The problem was that Sara's abdominal CT scan showed that her shunt tubing was sitting in a pocket of pus. Neurosurgical evaluation of this situation was imperative, but there was no pediatric neurosurgeon at the hospital where Sara was being treated. For this reason, Sara was transferred to Children's Hospital Los Angeles (CHLA).

As a fellow at CHLA, having completed my neuro-surgery residency training, I had privileges to manage patients independently as an attending neurosurgeon. On many nights and weekends, when patients came in who needed urgent interventions, I operated on them without my faculty supervisors present. I always first called my faculty supervisor to discuss the cases. Sara came in on a weekend when I was on call, and I went to the Emergency Department to evaluate her. I knew that antibiotics would never fully clear the infection in her abdomen with the shunt tubing in place, as the shunt was a foreign body now colonized by bacteria. So, the shunt needed to be removed from her abdomen. But Sara was presumed to be dependent upon her shunt, so it could not simply be removed—or she could get very sick quickly from increased pressure in the brain and even die. There were two options: (1) remove the abdominal portion of the shunt only and let the tubing drain into a bag temporarily until the infection cleared and a new shunt could be safely placed, or (2) remove the entire shunt—from head to abdomen—and place a catheter to drain fluid from the brain into a bag until a new shunt could be safely placed. In order to determine which of these options was the correct one, I needed to know whether the infection was confined to Sara's abdomen or if it had traveled along the shunt tubing to Sara's brain. I "tapped" the shunt—placing a small needle through the scalp into her shunt valve to sample the cerebrospinal fluid (CSF) in her brain. When the laboratory reported that her CSF was infected with gram-negative bacteria that later turned out to be Escherichia coli—a common bacteria found in the intestines—I knew that her entire shunt had to be removed. I called my faculty supervisor, Dr. J. Gordon McComb, who completely agreed and advised me to proceed.

There were two potential hazards to removing Sara's shunt. First, her ventricles—the fluid spaces within her brain—were relatively small because Sara's shunt was working properly to drain CSF from her brain to her abdomen. This meant that when I removed the catheter, it could be tricky to put the new catheter in the right place. But I had placed such catheters successfully in many patients with ventricles smaller than Sara's, and her ventricles looked reasonably accessible. Second, the neurosurgeon who had placed her shunt when she was a baby had used an outdated catheter that was risky to remove. Most shunt catheters are straight tubes that have little holes in the first few centimeters of tubing that allow CSF to enter. Sara's catheter additionally had "flanges"—little pieces of silicon that extended around the catheter tip. Flanged catheters were designed in the hope that the outpouchings would prevent the catheter holes from becoming occluded by debris or choroid plexus—a specialized tissue found in the ventricles that produces much of our CSF. In reality, it was found that rather than preventing shunt occlusion, flanged catheters often become stuck to the choroid plexus or brain and cause bleeding when removed. For this reason, they are rarely (if ever) used today. But, at that moment, I was stuck between a rock and a hard place. If I left the infected shunt catheter in place, Sara could develop meningitis that could cause death or severe disability. If I removed the flanged catheter, bleeding could occur that could damage her brain. Plus, her small ventricles made catheter malposition at least a possibility. I knew that there was no real choice—the shunt had to be removed in its entirety.

Before the surgery, I explained the risks of surgery to Sara's mother—spending extra time discussing the added risks caused by Sara's small ventricles and the flanged catheter. Her mother was worried about her daughter and distraught by the delay in diagnosing the appendicitis at the outside hospital. She seemed to understand everything I was saying, and she signed a consent form giving permission for surgery to proceed.

At surgery, I opened the prior scalp incision and disconnected the catheter going into the brain from the shunt valve. I easily removed the shunt valve and all the tubing going into the abdomen via this single incision. Now it was time to remove the catheter going into the ventricle of the brain. I was worried that it would be stuck—making it more likely for bleeding to occur with removal—but it actually came out easily. I breathed a sigh of relief. However, when I placed the new catheter down the same tract, the CSF that emerged—which is typically clear like water—was quite bloody. So, I did what I had been taught to do in this situation and had done a number of times previously. I attached a syringe and slowly irrigated ten milliliters of normal saline into the brain, then slowly withdrew the same amount of bloody fluid. I repeated that maneuver numerous times over around twenty minutes. Ten milliliters in, ten milliliters out. I patiently waited for the bleeding to stop and the fluid to clear, which it eventually did. I then secured the catheter to the skin with sutures, connected it to a drainage bag, and confirmed that it was dripping clear fluid into the bag. I then closed the scalp with sutures.

Sara emerged normally from anesthesia and was brought to the recovery room. I went to the waiting room and told Sara's mother that we had removed the shunt but there had been some bleeding from the catheter removal—as I had warned her—but that it had cleared with irrigation, and I expected Sara to likely be fine. Shortly thereafter, I went to examine Sara. I knew something was wrong when I asked her to lift up both of her arms and she did so, but her right arm was considerably weaker than her left arm. She lifted her left arm up briskly and high and easily held it in the air. But she struggled to lift her right arm against gravity. She would lift it about halfway as high as the left arm and then it would fall down onto the bed. I ordered an urgent CT of her brain to find out why. The CT scan showed—to my dismay—that the new catheter that I thought I had placed down the same tract into the ventricle was actually approximately one centimeter too lateral and was sitting in the basal ganglia, an area of the brain involved in motor function among other things. Next to the catheter was a cavitation that included both blood and fluid. When I thought during surgery that I was irrigating out blood from the ventricle, I had actually been irrigating in and out of the brain tissue right next to the ventricle. There was no way for me to know this during the surgery, as catheter placement is always a "blind" procedure—performed without direct visualization of the target.

Still, I felt terrible. I had placed hundreds of shunt catheters before, and I had never caused a new neurological problem. I went back to Sara's mother, showed her the CT scan, and told her how sorry I was that this complication occurred. I told her that we needed to go back to the operating room to reposition the catheter, as it was currently draining fluid but was in the wrong place and I did not want to risk acute symptoms from hydrocephalus. After obtaining consent from Sara's mother, I went back to the operating room with Sara. Guided by the new CT scan, I removed the catheter and placed a new one in a more medial direction into the ventricle, as documented by another CT scan after the second surgery. Unfortunately, Sara's new right-sided weakness persisted.

Over the next few weeks, Sara received antibiotics and the infection cleared. To our team's surprise—as this happens uncommonly—we never needed to replace her shunt, which was great news. After draining CSF for a few days into the bag, we took advantage of Sara's shunt being externalized to clamp it and monitor her intracranial pressure and symptoms. With the drain clamped, her pressure remained normal and she had no headache or other new symptoms. A CT scan showed that her ventricles remained small, so we removed the drain permanently. She then went to CHLA's inpatient rehabilitation unit where she received intensive physical and occupational therapy, and her right-sided weakness gradually improved. She could now lift up her right arm much better and grasp objects. She could walk, but her walking was somewhat awkward because her right leg was weaker than the left. Unfortunately, she never fully recovered the function that she had lost.

During Sara's hospitalization and rehabilitation stays, I visited her frequently and spent as much extra time with her and her mother as I could. Each time I saw her, I relived her surgery in my mind and wished that I had not placed that catheter too laterally. Dr. McComb graciously comforted me, reminding me that the only neurosurgeon who never put a shunt catheter in the wrong place was one who didn't place shunt catheters. I appreciated Dr. McComb's support, but it did not completely comfort me. I knew that it had been my hands that had caused a new problem in an adorable little girl that would affect her for the rest of her life. I felt immense guilt. The two things that gave me comfort were the fact that Sara was gaining strength week by week and that I had a great relationship with her mother—or so I thought. Her mother greeted me warmly each time I came to visit Sara and frequently told me how much Sara was improving. Soon after Sara was discharged home from rehab, I finished my fellowship at

CHLA and moved to Miami to join the faculty at the University of Miami. I said goodbye to Sara and her mother and thought that I was leaving things on great terms.

Approximately two years later, I was sitting in my office when my administrative assistant knocked on my door and told me that there was a man at the front desk with a manila envelope that only I could sign for. When I opened up the envelope and began reading, I was dumbstruck. The envelope contained a summons (judicial notification) informing me that Sara's family had filed a medical malpractice lawsuit. There were several doctors named, along with the hospital, but mine was the first name on the list.

I felt an immediate rush of so many emotions. The first one was fear about the implications of this lawsuit. What would this mean for my professional reputation? Who would find out about this? Would this make it harder for me to get a new job in the future? The second was sadness about my relationship with Sara's mother. I had done my very best to care for her daughter in a very high-risk situation given her small ventricles and flanged catheter. After the complication had occurred, I had poured my heart into both optimizing her care and comforting her mother. I felt blindsided by what felt like a personal attack despite my best efforts.

My dominant emotion over the months that followed was anger. Depositions, phone calls, and meetings with my attorney took countless hours away from my already busy and stressful life, and I resented every minute of it. I was certain that Sara's complication could have happened to any neurosurgeon unfortunate enough to be placed in the predicament of having to remove a flanged catheter stuck to the brain or choroid plexus. I would never minimize the implications for Sara, and I felt terrible about her right-sided weakness that occurred following my surgery. But this weakness was the result of a complication—very different from medical malpractice, which is defined by deviation from the current standard of care. It is stressful enough to perform neurosurgical procedures. It felt completely unfair to be punished in this way when I had managed Sara exactly as is taught in neurosurgery textbooks and how I had been trained by my mentors.

I was advised by several neurosurgery colleagues who had been through legal cases before that I should try to settle the case as soon as possible. They warned me that depositions and meetings were annoying enough, but that going through a trial was not only incredibly anxiety-provoking, but it wreaked havoc from a logistical standpoint. Trials can last for weeks, and their dates constantly get changed. It is complicated enough to schedule surgeries; what would I tell families when I had to cancel surgeries to go to trial? Should I tell them the real reason? I feared that if I did so, parents of potential future patients might decide that they didn't want me to take care of their child. Despite the advice I received, I could not come to terms with agreeing to settle the case. Settling the case was essentially an admission that I had committed malpractice, which I had not. I simply could not bring myself to do this. I resolved to refuse to settle the case under any circumstance regardless of whatever hassle and anxiety awaited me.

I was so lucky to be assigned an extraordinary attorney for my defense—Robert McKenna. Robert is as passionate about defending physicians who are wrongly sued as I am about taking care of patients. Everything about Robert gave me confidence and hope when I really needed it. Robert fully supported my insistence on fighting the lawsuit to the bitter end and refusing to settle. He told me that while he could not guarantee what a jury would do, he felt that the odds were strongly in my favor because—based on his experience and what he was told by the pediatric neurosurgeon serving as expert witness—I had not actually deviated from the standard of care. He was so detail-oriented, analyzing every line of the medical record over and over again and asking me the most thoughtful questions. The more I got to know him, the more he served not only as my attorney but also as a friend and a therapist of sorts. He told me not to take the lawsuit personally. Sara's mother was financially strapped and raising eight children on her own, as the children's father was incarcerated. Robert said that sometimes the origins of a lawsuit are related to financial considerations rather than any ill feelings Sara's mother may have toward me. He told me to view the case in more transactional terms, and this was helpful to me. Moreover, he seemed as angry as I was that I was being sued, and he even told me that if—God forbid—his own child had a neurosurgical condition, he would not hesitate in turning to me. I really needed to hear this in a moment during which I felt so vulnerable.

Going through the trial was one of the worst experiences of my life. I had to leave my practice in Miami and travel to Los Angeles for two weeks—counted as vacation—and reschedule multiple clinics and surgeries. I was so stressed that I slept no more than two hours in any of the nights I spent in the hotel in LA. The whole courtroom experience seemed very staged. Robert gave me instructions on every detail down to what I should wear. He told me to wear a white shirt each day with a plain dark suit and bland tie. I needed to make sure that none of these clothes were fancy brands to avoid looking flashy. He told me to wear a simple Casio watch and my wedding ring but no other jewelry. He told me that my wife, Amy, who wanted to come to the trial to support me, should not attend. Her presence would potentially make it look like I was nervous enough to bring my wife, which would imply that I was guilty.

During the trial, the plaintiff's attorney and his expert witnesses tried to portray me as the devil himself. They also tried to blame me for Sara's preexisting medical problems related to her prematurity. Preoperatively, Sara had language and developmental delays. In an effort to get the highest possible payout from the jury, the plaintiff's attorney and his expert witness claimed that Sara would need therapies to address these issues for the rest of her life without stating that these problems preceded the surgery. The single worst session was the testimony of the neurosurgeon hired by the plaintiff's attorney as an expert witness. I was so offended that a neurosurgeon would actually testify that my care for Sara constituted medical malpractice, and I was so curious to hear what she would actually say.

What I heard was infuriating. The neurosurgeon—a practicing pediatric neurosurgeon from another state—said that she agreed with my judgment that Sara's infected shunt had to be removed and replaced by an externalized drain. She acknowledged that shunt catheters can be challenging to place in children with small ventricles and that catheter malposition does not constitute malpractice. But she claimed that the fluid next to the catheter on the postoperative CT proved that I had irrigated more fluid into the brain than I had removed. This, she claimed, was below the standard of care and was the cause of Sara's postoperative weakness. But this simply wasn't true! I had removed exactly ten milliliters following every ten-milliliter infusion of normal saline until the blood had cleared. I, too, had been puzzled by the fluid collection on the postoperative CT, but it must have been caused by a mixture of blood products and CSF. I felt vindicated when Robert's skillful cross-examination made the neurosurgery expert witness appear flustered and vindictive. I wondered to myself what was the motivation for this neurosurgeon to agree to be an expert witness in this case. Money is the obvious answer, as neurosurgeons who serve as expert witnesses are often paid large sums of money—sometimes over $1,000 per hour. But neurosurgeons are paid very well, and why was it worth it to her to make this extra money by incorrectly claiming to know what happened during a challenging case that she did not observe?

My own testimony was emotional but much less painful because I felt as though I was regaining control of the narrative—and I felt empowered because my version of events was the truth. The cross-examination portion was frustrating, as the plaintiff's attorney asked me the same questions over and over again, with slight twists, trying to goad me into appearing angry or saying something stupid. Next came the defense expert witness—a very senior and prominent pediatric neurosurgeon. I was so relieved when he testified that what had happened in Sara's case not only could not be described as malpractice but had happened to him several times in his career. I felt so grateful to him for this testimony, but I also took mental note that he, too, was earning thousands of dollars. There were so many things that seemed flawed about this whole legal process.

At the end of the trial, the jury took only a few hours before emerging. As the judge read the jury's unanimous verdict—that I had not committed malpractice—I breathed a huge sigh of relief. But I did not feel any sense of triumph. I felt exhausted and emotionally depleted. I looked over at Sara's mother and I felt sad for her and for

Sara (who was not in the courtroom at that moment). There were no winners in this case—we were all losers.

Surgical complications cause tremendous heartache—especially for the patient and the patient's family but also for the surgeon. The only positive that comes out of them is the learning experience that hopefully prevents the same complication from happening again. I saw many surgical disasters during my residency training and fellowship, both at top programs in our country. When I finished my fellowship in 2004, I felt ready and qualified to tackle the most difficult surgical cases, and I did so with great confidence. But there is no question in my mind that I am a better doctor and surgeon now than I was in 2004. I am more skilled technically, and I am also more humble. I have learned from my own complications and from those of my colleagues. Every year that goes by, I appreciate more and more how fragile and unpredictable the human body—and especially the nervous system—can be.

One of the most memorable neurosurgery conferences I ever attended was an annual meeting of the American Society of Pediatric Neurosurgeons (ASPN) a few years ago. Those at the meeting were all attending pediatric neurosurgeons, many of whom were very senior and among the most respected pediatric neurosurgeons in the world. Each neurosurgeon was asked to present the worst complication of his or her career. This is an uncommon dynamic, as most medical conferences focus on scientific research or new approaches to treating diseases. This session, on the other hand, was like group therapy! After some presentations, colleagues came up and gave the speaker a hug or offered supportive pats on the back. I realized that even the most admired senior neurosurgeons have had their own disastrous complications. This conference not only provided wisdom, enabling me to learn from the complications of my colleagues, but it allowed a measure of healing for me regarding patients like James and Sara. It was so helpful for me to know that not only am I not alone, but that not one of my talented colleagues from around the world had avoided serious complications in their careers.

Because of the massive impact that surgical complications have on our patients, we are morally obligated to do everything in our power to prevent them. In particular, surgeons must have the humility to know that we do not know everything. We are humans, prone to error. For this reason, group discussions about cases prior to surgery are extremely beneficial. One of the first things I implemented when I became the director of the division of pediatric neurosurgery at my medical center was a weekly conference in which all surgical cases for the coming week are presented. Our team has four pediatric neurosurgeons, and we mostly trained at different institutions. We each bring a unique perspective. All four of us attend this conference along with an outstanding neuroradiologist who provides her perspective on MRI scans, CT scans, and other imaging studies our patients undergo prior to surgery. Because we are an academic institution, there are residents and students in attendance as well.

If you attended these conferences, you would be surprised how often my pediatric neurosurgery partners—each of whom is an outstanding physician and surgeon—disagree with me and with each other on the best approach to any given case. On a number of occasions, after hearing the opinions of my colleagues and our neuroradiologist, I have changed my surgical approach. Similarly, there are many times that I have convinced my colleagues to do something differently. On a few occasions, I or one of my partners have canceled scheduled surgical cases—even on the same day of surgery when the patient and family have arrived prepared to proceed. It takes humility to go out and tell a family, after a long discussion in the office and much buildup to the moment of surgery, that your partners have convinced you that the operation should be delayed or canceled. But humility is required in medicine, and it is acquired by the challenging experience of living through awful complications with patients and families and desperately wanting to avoid bad outcomes.

6

Pulled in Many Directions: A Day in the Life of a Pediatric Neurosurgeon

On a typical Wednesday morning a few years ago, I was in the middle of a delicate surgery to remove a brain tumor in an eleven-month-old boy named Mohammed. The surgery was going extremely well. I had just completed the tumor resection, and I was grateful that I had been able to remove the tumor without much blood loss in this very fragile baby. All that was left was to close the dura, reattach the piece of the skull that I had removed to gain access to the tumor and close the scalp incision. I had no other surgeries scheduled that day, and I was looking forward to eating lunch and then catching up on some research projects. I am never hungry when I am performing the critical portion of operations because I am so focused on the task at hand. Now that the critical portion was completed and the closure was about to begin, I felt my stomach growling.

My cell phone rang, and I asked the circulating nurse in the operating room to answer it. I frowned underneath my mask because this was the fourth time my phone had gone off in the last hour. "That phone is a weapon," I mumbled to myself as I so often do when my phone rings during surgery. One of my favorite things about being in surgery is that I am focused on a single task with none of the constant daily distractions that we all struggle with in the modern world such as texts, emails, and telemarketers. The operating room is often a haven from phone calls and emails, and I was annoyed that this peaceful space was being disrupted yet again. I wish that I could turn my phone off during surgeries but this is not possible because of additional emergencies that might require immediate decisions.

When the nurse heard the words coming from the person on the other end of the phone, she quickly walked toward me and said, "I think you need to take this one." She put the phone to my ear, and I listened to the neurosurgery resident on the other end. She told me about a life-threatening emergency at MD Anderson Cancer Center, two blocks from where I was currently operating at Children's Memorial Hermann Hospital. She quickly rattled off, "Felipe had a seizure and came in through the emergency room. He was lethargic, so they got a CT scan. There is a huge hemorrhage in the previous tumor resection cavity with mass effect and midline shift. They are transferring him to the pediatric intensive care unit." After asking a few questions about the CT scan and Felipe's condition, I instructed her to book Felipe for emergency surgery to remove the blood clot. I told her to get consent from Felipe's parents and to tell them that I couldn't speak to them myself at the moment because I was in the middle of another surgery. I asked her to reassure them that we would arrange for an operating room to be prepared right away, and that I would be there as soon as the operating room at MD Anderson was ready.

I knew I had about forty-five minutes until the next operating room would be ready. In those forty-five minutes, I needed to finish the current surgery, talk to Mohammed's parents, and then race over to MD Anderson. In some situations, I might have asked one of my partners to help since I simply can't be in two operating rooms in different hospitals at the same time. But I knew Felipe's parents very well, and given everything we had been through together, I knew that they would be deeply disappointed and very anxious if I didn't perform his surgery myself.

Felipe was a five-year-old boy who had started having headaches about a year before and was found to have a large tumor that had bled in the left frontal lobe of his brain. It turned out to be a very aggressive cancer called a sarcoma. Despite surgery to completely remove the tumor, radiation therapy, and chemotherapy, the tumor kept coming back, and it always bled when it recurred. His parents had come from South America for me to perform the initial operation, and they had not been back home since. After several surgeries and so many difficult discussions, he and his parents felt like family to me. I had to be the one to perform this surgery.

Of course, I also felt equal responsibility to the family of Mohammed, whose operation I was in the middle of performing. I closed the dura and skull as quickly as possible, and the last skin suture was placed about thirty-five minutes later. I left the assisting neurosurgery resident to put on the bandage and gave him instructions regarding postoperative orders. I sprinted out of the operating room and spoke to Mohammed's parents, sharing the good news that the surgery was a big success. I then raced to MD Anderson, arriving just as Felipe was wheeled into the operating room. I changed my scrubs while simultaneously shoving a banana and four spoonfuls of peanut butter into my mouth, and I walked into the operating room just as the team was ready for me to position Felipe for surgery. Two hours later, after successfully removing a huge blood clot and saving Felipe's life, I sat down with his parents in the recovery room to have an extended discussion about the surgery and next steps. I apologized for not talking to them in person before the surgery, but they graciously understood.

Thankfully, situations like this don't happen every day. I am often needed in more than one place at a time, but I am rarely needed in two operating rooms simultaneously. When there are two simultaneous emergencies, I always figure out a way to manage the situation, and I can count on my partners to jump in and help. But I am often struck by the fact that the parents of each child have no idea that anything is going on with any other child but their own. I try my best to make every patient and family feel as though they are my only priority, but I sometimes wonder how families would feel if they knew how many patients I often manage simultaneously.

Patients and families only see a brief glimpse of my day when I meet them in the clinic, emergency room, or in the hospital wards. My interactions with them are often at odd hours—very early in the morning, late at night, or on weekends and holidays. "Are you always here?" "Do you ever go home?" These are common questions that I hear from families. The answer to the first question is "no" and the answer to the second question is "yes," but I do work very hard and spend many hours at work. Additionally, I feel very lucky to have a wonderful family and home life.

Because pediatric neurosurgeons are often called to evaluate life-or-death emergencies, children's hospitals must have a pediatric neurosurgeon on call twenty-four hours a day, seven days a week, three hundred and sixty-five days a year. For most of the past ten years, I have shared call with two partners, so I have been on call one-third of the time. When on call, I must be reachable at all times, and I always stay within a fifteen-minute drive from the hospital. Even when I am not on call, I am often called by referring doctors or colleagues with questions regarding an existing or new patient. So, I never turn off my phone, including on vacation. Essentially, the only time I am not reachable is when I am on an airplane. While most people silence their phones at night before they go to sleep, I never do so. I get annoyed with friends or family members who forget this and call or text too late when I am sleeping. My close friends and family know never to call or text me after about 9:30 P.M., as I might have been up much of the night before or trying to get rest the night before a big surgery.

Some call nights are quiet. Sometimes I don't receive a single phone call. On other nights, I am bombarded with call after call all night long or have to come to the hospital for one or more emergencies. Most of the time, when I come in at night, it's for an emergency surgery. At other times, I come to the hospital to talk to a family about a new serious diagnosis or to give the horrible news that nothing can be done to save a child's life after a horrible trauma or brain bleed. My dream job would be one in which neurosurgical emergencies only happened during daylight hours, but no such job exists. I am, therefore, almost always at least a little sleep-deprived. I feel the sleep deprivation much more at home than at work. At work, especially when I am performing surgery, adrenaline and focus prevent me from feeling tired. When I eventually get home though, I am sometimes completely exhausted.

My wife, kids, and friends frequently make fun of me for falling asleep at dinner tables, on couches, and during movies and TV shows, but I don't mind. I love my job and my life, and I always remind myself that it's never as bad as my time at Jamaica Hospital.

On weekends when I am on call, I typically "make rounds" (visit with each patient currently in the hospital with a neurosurgical problem) on Saturday and Sunday mornings and then only come back to the hospital for emergencies. On many weekends when I am not on call, I still come to the hospital to check on my patients. Weekdays are filled with many different activities depending upon the day. If I am on call, my alarm is set for 5:20 A.M. so that I can arrive at the hospital at 6:00 A.M. to make rounds with my team. Together with a neurosurgery resident and/or pediatric neurosurgery fellow, physician assistant, and medical students rotating on our service, I check on hospitalized patients. We meet in the pediatric intensive care unit where we gather around a computer and first review new imaging studies and other pertinent test results. Then, we see between ten and twenty-five hospitalized patients. Typically, we finish rounds by around 7:00 A.M.

On many days after rounds, I have academic teaching conferences. These include lectures on neurosurgery topics, our team's pediatric neurosurgery/neuroradiology conference, Morbidity and Mortality conference, and lectures by visiting professors. On some days, typically one-and-a-half days per week, I see outpatients in the clinic (typically between thirty and forty patients per day). On most other days, I am in the operating room performing surgeries. When I am not operating or seeing patients in the hospital or clinic, my time is spent catching up on documentation for medical records, returning phone calls or emails about patients, and working on research projects. Many hours are also spent going to endless meetings because of my role as director of our division of pediatric neurosurgery.

When I am not physically in the hospital or clinic, I can be found in my academic office trying to catch up on replying to the one hundred to two hundred emails I receive each day. When I return to my desk after an eight-hour surgery, my inbox is always filled with emails, many of which are from individuals who expect an immediate response. These emails come from patients' parents, research colleagues and staff, my administrative assistant about logistical arrangements, families interested in our clinical trials from around the world, students who want to shadow me, neurosurgeons who want to come for a fellowship—and the list goes on. Life is a constant battle to catch up on emails, and this battle is never won. I think that this sentiment is common to almost every profession in the digital age.

Besides surgical complications, which cause the most stress, the next most stressful thing for me is being needed in more than one place at the same time. So many times, I have felt terrible for leaving or canceling a meeting because of a neurosurgical emergency. I feel incredibly stressed when an emergency happens during my clinic. I want my team to provide great service for all patients, and I feel horrible about leaving patients waiting for a long time while I attend to the sickest patient. It's bad enough that their parents had to take off work, drive to the medical center, pay for parking, etc. I am fortunate to have dedicated partners who are always willing to jump in and help, but I often find myself more reluctant to accept help than I should be.

It has struck me over the past decade that there is a new focus among many young professionals—almost to the point of obsession—with wellness and work-life balance. Many work conferences in different professional fields include sessions on such topics. It is my impression that compared to decades ago, intruding on coworkers' personal time with work requests is more frowned upon than previously. Many workers have outgoing email messages that state that they don't check email after hours or on the weekend. Email application programs ask if you want to schedule your email to send during business hours to be more respectful. Undoubtedly, as digital communication has increased, the need for these guardrails has increased. However, what I believe many aspiring young people struggle to understand is that certain jobs like pediatric neurosurgery require that there be no guardrails when the job is being performed at the highest level. If your child had an emergent brain bleed in the middle of the night, would you prefer that the surgeon who had operated on your child twice and knew your child's history intimately take care of it, or that a stranger do it? Such a commitment to this level of care results in a lifestyle with real limitations and no truly protected time, which our culture generally discourages. I do wonder what effect this will have on the quality of pediatric neurosurgical care for the next generation. I wonder if subspecialists like neurosurgeons will wind up performing fewer surgical cases during their residency and thereafter and thus be less skilled. I also wonder whether too many doctors will adopt a shift worker mentality rather than owning their patient's care regardless of personal inconvenience.

Patience is not my strong suit—both because of my innate makeup and because I am pulled in so many directions. My patience is tested every day in one way or another. It is tested in the operating room when waiting for a patient to get to the room or for an anesthesiologist to start an IV line—which can be quite challenging in babies and young children. It is tested during surgical procedures when I am supervising residents doing things slower than I would. I feel impatient when I am trapped in endless meetings, some of which are inefficient. I try so hard to be patient with families, understanding that any visit to a pediatric neurosurgeon is immensely stressful for parents. Most of the time, I think I do a pretty good job, but sometimes I fall short. I must admit feeling annoyed when the same question is asked over and over again. I sometimes have to hold myself back from saying, "Were you not listening when I answered that question twice already within the past ten minutes?" I also feel frustrated when I have just had a forty-five-minute discussion with a parent and at the very end, he or she asks if I can have the same conversation with another family member. On the other hand, I feel immense gratitude when families recognize how busy I am and go out of their way to be respectful of my time. At the end of the day, I am fully aware that I must strive to make every parent feel as though their child is my only patient. I try my best to do so, but I am not perfect.

There are uncommon situations, such as when I am out of town or have an important family event such as a wedding, when I simply cannot attend to my patients, and must rely on my partners. But in general, when I have a patient who is in the hospital and has a worrisome problem, everything else in my life is on hold. My family and friends understand that I may need to leave a dinner or other activity at any moment. And there have certainly been plenty of days over the years when, sadly, I didn't get to see my kids all day. Other days I barely make it in time to spend a few minutes with my kids. I recall one day around seven years ago when I got home at 8:30 P.M. after a busy day that included three surgeries. When I got home, my wife, Amy, told me that our seven-year-old son, Benjamin, was already asleep. I was sad because I had left in the morning before he was awake and didn't make it in time to see him at night, either. But Amy had just put Dalia, my nine-year-old daughter, to bed, and she told me that Dalia wasn't yet sleeping and I could run in quickly to say goodnight. When I walked into Dalia's room, the lights were off but she was still awake. I jumped into Dalia's bed. She gave me a big hug and said, "Oh my God, I thought it was a burglar but then I realized it was Daddy and my heart leaped!" Hearing these words was the sweetest thing in the world, and I remember them to this day.

Thankfully, on most days when I get home from work I can spend quality time with my family. At this point, in fact, my teenage kids stay up later than I do on most nights. I have never missed a family birthday celebration or any other important family event. I am lucky to have a wonderful wife, who is a busy physician herself, and two amazing children. Despite my demanding career, I am proud to be a 50/50 parent who is equally engaged in all matters related to our kids. My advice to those considering demanding careers such as neurosurgery who are also passionate about being truly engaged as a partner and/or parent is twofold. First, set realistic expectations. Don't tell anyone that you will definitely be home for an event or make it to your kid's soccer game if you might not make it. Second, when you are home, be as present as you possibly can. Answer work-related phone calls but try to otherwise be off your phone. Be the first to jump up to clean the dishes or change a dirty diaper and the first to get down on the floor to play with your young child no matter how tired you are. When you can't spend the quantity of time that you wish you could with your family, make sure that the time you do have is truly high quality.

I encourage medical students considering a career in neurosurgery to understand the challenges of this road but to also know that it is possible to be a neurosurgeon and still have a wonderful family life—as long as you are surrounded by family members who understand the unique nature of this commitment and the inability to ever truly disconnect from patient care. My hope is that there will be young people in the future who embrace this level of commitment with pride, for the good of future children with serious neurosurgical illness.

Bicycles, Bullets, and Beaten Babies: Keeping Our Children Safe

A two-year-old girl was playing with her mother on her parents' bed. All of a sudden, without any warning, the little girl leaped off the bed before her mom had a chance to catch her. She slammed her head against the hard wooden bedframe. The little girl did not lose consciousness, but she was screaming her head off and had significant swelling of her scalp where she had smacked her head. As a pediatric neurosurgeon working at a busy trauma center, I had been consulted on patients like this child countless times. In the overwhelming majority of head traumas from low heights where the child has not lost consciousness, there are no meaningful consequences for the child. A small minority, however, can have depressed skull fractures or even life-threatening blood clots that require emergent surgery. But there was something very different about this particular case. This little girl was my daughter.

My wife, Amy, called me immediately, and I could hear the stress in her voice along with our daughter, Dalia, screaming bloody murder in the background. I told Amy to get in the car immediately and bring Dalia to the hospital. When they arrived ten minutes later, Dalia was wide awake and neurologically normal but still screaming at the top of her lungs. When I moved her beautiful red curls out of the way, I could see the impressive scalp swelling where she had hit her head, likely from a blood clot underneath her skin. I carried Dalia in my arms directly to the CT scanner. She was terrified of the CT scan, but we strapped her down to take pictures of her brain and skull that would take only two minutes but seem like eternity.

I tend to stay calm in pressured situations, and I certainly stay calm on the outside. I reassured Amy that the overwhelming statistical odds were that the CT would show nothing at all, and I knew that this was true. As I waited for the images to come up, though, I felt my heart rate increase. I couldn't keep my mind from wandering to the unthinkable situation I might find myself in just two minutes from now. So many thoughts and questions raced through my head all at once. What if the tables were about to turn, and I was about to be the father of a patient needing brain surgery rather than the child's neurosurgeon? What if my precious daughter had a big blood clot shifting over her brain? What if she looked fine now but was about to deteriorate? Which of my partners would I trust the most to do the operation, and which were available? And, most important, was she going to be okay?

Thankfully, Dalia's CT scan showed no abnormality other than a scalp bruise. There was no skull fracture and not a drop of blood in her brain. Amy and I breathed a huge collective sigh of relief. In hindsight, the unforgettable experience of having my daughter rushed to the hospital with a potential head injury gave me a small taste of the agony that the parents of my patients go through. Amy was tortured by guilt because this had happened under her watch. I felt terrible for Amy, as I knew that this could easily have happened under my watch, too. My reassurance that I had seen things like this happen countless times to wonderful and attentive parents did little to comfort her. On many occasions since that day, I have told the story of Dalia's trip to the emergency room to crying parents overwhelmed by guilt after dropping their baby or not being there in time to catch their toddler who fell from a low height. It was definitely good for me to experience—relatively early in my career—the anxiety that the parents of my patients go through when waiting for the results of an imaging study. I was forced to experience for myself what it feels like for your heart to be racing as pictures are taken of your child's brain that could alter the trajectory of your child's life—and therefore your own life, too—forever.

The scary thing about head trauma is that freak accidents can occur even during the most innocuous activities and result in tragedy. Believe it or not, I witnessed a child die from playing Duck, Duck, Goose. In November 2021, I was consulted emergently on a ten-year-old girl who had been playing Duck, Duck, Goose at school during recess. While running around the circle of kids, she had a head-on-head collision with a classmate. When she went home, she told her parents that her head was hurting, and her parents took her to the pediatrician's office. The pediatrician checked her out and found nothing wrong on clinical examination. When the family got home from the pediatrician's office, the child took a nap while the parents went shopping at Walmart (with the child's grandparents staying with the child). When the parents got back from Walmart, they could not arouse their daughter and they called 911. When the child arrived at our hospital, a CT scan showed a massive hemorrhage in her brain, and we could not save her because she was clinically brain-dead. To be clear, this was a highly unusual event, and I would not recommend that any parent forbid their child from playing Duck, Duck, Goose. But it illustrates our collective fragility and vulnerability to random, crazy events.

While freak accidents can happen to any child or adult, so many of the devastating injuries that I treat on a daily basis are doubly tragic because they are completely preventable. One prime example of this is head trauma in children riding bicycles without protective helmets. Numerous research studies have documented that bicycle helmets significantly reduce the odds of a serious or fatal head injury.[1] I have cared for so many children who require emergent surgeries or have permanent disabilities or even die after falling off their bicycle or when their bicycle gets hit by a car. In the twenty-six years that I have taken care of neurosurgical trauma patients, I cannot recall a single child wearing a helmet who suffered a devastating head injury.

When I was a child riding my bike to school each day—without a helmet—bicycle helmets were not in widespread use. In fact, I don't recall ever seeing any kid on a bike wearing a helmet throughout my childhood. These days, as the protective effect of helmets has become clear, helmets are used by many children and adults although they clearly have not been universally adopted. In discussions with parents whose children are hospitalized after bicycle injuries, it has become evident to me that some parents—especially those with lower incomes and less education—have not been adequately informed about the importance of helmet use. Other children don't have helmets because of the cost. A good bicycle helmet currently costs around forty dollars, which is affordable to most families but not viewed as a critical purchase by disadvantaged families who are watching every penny, particularly if they have more than one child. Some parents of teenagers tell me that they bought helmets for their kids, but their kids refuse to wear them. As the father of two teenagers, I fully understand that parents don't have full control over their kids' decisions. But head trauma without a helmet can be a life-or-death situation, and I suspect that some parents who don't force their children to use them don't fully realize this—or they would be stricter on this issue. While it may be too late in some circumstances, I do feel the need to educate parents about helmet use at this crucial teaching moment. If not now, then when? I urge parents to teach their children about the importance of wearing a helmet every time they get on a bicycle with no exceptions. Same goes for ATVs, scooters, hoverboards, and motorized bikes. As kids get older and are riding around unsupervised, I advise parents to consider taking away the bicycle or other recreational device if their child refuses to wear a helmet.

The most common cause of head and spine injuries in adolescents and adults is motor vehicle accidents.[2] In the coming years, motor vehicle accident injuries and deaths will hopefully decrease in frequency due to more wide-spread seatbelt use, airbags, and electronic safety features in new car models. However, so far these safety features have not come close to eliminating devastating injuries and deaths. I urge caretakers to drive safely and to make sure that children are in age-appropriate car seats or boosters. I emphasize seatbelt use, including in the back seat. Too often, people who don't wear seatbelts don't walk out of hospitals—they are wheeled or carried. Anecdotally, it seems to me that the most common seatbelt not to be fastened is in the back middle seat. I vividly recall one child who suffered a severe traumatic brain injury from a motor vehicle accident. She was one of five passengers, and she was sitting in the back middle seat when the car was involved in a high-speed motor vehicle crash. She was the only passenger not wearing a seatbelt—and the only passenger who was injured. She spent three weeks in the intensive care unit and six weeks in inpatient rehabilitation. The other four walked away from the accident unscathed.

I am asked frequently about the safety of participation in various sports both by parents of patients with various neurosurgical conditions and by friends whose children have no medical conditions. There is no sport or activity that is completely free of risk. At any given moment, a child is safer sitting on a couch than on a sports field, but the health and emotional benefits of exercise and youth athletic participation are clearly recognized and generally outweigh the risks of injury. As the father of a boy who is serious about soccer and plays many hours each week, the single scariest sports injury that I have seen was an eight-year-old boy who died after a head-on-head collision at a soccer game. Several hours after the game, the boy started vomiting and then quickly had altered mental status. His parents called 911, and an ambulance came right away, but he was brain-dead by the time he made it to our hospital.

A CT scan showed a massive epidural hematoma—a bleed between the skull and the covering of the brain just like Garrett's in chapter one—but he arrived at our hospital too late for surgery to save him.

After this happened, I asked myself whether I should allow my son to play soccer. I was already concerned about the risks of heading a soccer ball, my least favorite part of the sport. US Club Soccer, a national youth soccer organization, recommends no heading in children under ten and limited heading in children ages eleven and twelve,[3] but there is nothing magical that happens when you turn thirteen that protects the brain from the possible risks of heading a hard soccer ball repeatedly. My wife and I do allow our son to play soccer, but we make him wear a protective headband. Protective headbands made for soccer are approximately one-half inch thick and are easily fitted to the head with a Velcro strap. They are commercially available but used by very few soccer players. While there is no proof that they provide any definite protection, and they do nothing to diminish the impact of heading the ball, the headbands may minimize the impact of head-on-head collisions, and they make us feel better. Our son is the only kid in his youth soccer league or school team who wears a protective headband, as most parents don't even know about them. A few times, he has been teased by his teammates or even his coaches for wearing the headband, but he knows that he's not allowed to step on a soccer field without it.

I am often struck by the overwhelming importance that sports participation plays in the lives of so many kids. To be clear, I personally view athletics as having a hugely positive impact in the lives of children. I am an ex-athlete myself—I played water polo in high school and college. But occasionally, kids and their parents take sports so seriously that they lose perspective. I recall a freak injury that happened to a teenager during a baseball game. The boy was playing in the outfield, and he ran back to try to catch a ball that was hit deep in the outfield. As he was going for the ball, he slammed his head into a concrete post that was holding up the fence. He suffered an obvious depressed skull fracture in his forehead with injury to his underlying brain that required emergent surgery. I was dumbstruck when his parents asked me immediately after the surgery when he could return to practice and then over and over again whether this would ruin his baseball career, but they never once asked me if the injury would affect their son's school performance or cause any other type of impairment that would affect his life outside of baseball.

The single most common conversation I have both with patients' parents and with friends is about participation in tackle football. To be clear, this is a topic of great controversy, even among neurosurgeons. Some of my neurosurgery colleagues allow their own sons to play tackle football and argue that severe brain and spine injuries are relatively rare in youth football. Other neurosurgeons would never let their child participate in tackle football. I fall into the latter group. My first concern is the long-term impact of concussions, which are more common in tackle football than in most other sports. Chronic traumatic encephalopathy (CTE), a serious syndrome that includes behavior problems, cognitive decline, and even dementia, is caused by repetitive head trauma. CTE has been mostly prominently documented in professional football players who have died and undergone autopsy evaluation of their brains, but there are increasing reports of CTE in younger, nonprofessional athletes including teenagers.[4]

If the risks associated with repetitive head injuries are not enough, the risk of devastating neck injuries is the nail in the coffin for me. Over the course of my career, I have seen approximately ten kids—all teenagers—who have suffered permanent neurological impairment from a cervical spine injury that occurred while playing tackle football. Some of these kids are in wheelchairs for the rest of their lives. While youth players are instructed to never put their head down when they make a tackle, all it takes is one tackle with bad form—or landing on your head when being tackled—to risk an injury to the cervical spine that can cause permanent disability. Football is taken very seriously in the state of Texas where I live and in many other places, too. I tell parents that, statistically, the chances of their children making a living on Sundays playing in the NFL is tiny compared to the chance that they will earn a living using their brains from Monday to Friday, and they should think seriously about the risks before allowing participation in tackle football.

Despite my concerns about the safety of tackle football, I must confess that I am a season ticket holder to the NFL's Houston Texans. I completely recognize my own hypocrisy here. How can I spend money supporting a sport that I consider too dangerous to allow my own son to play? Each season I think about canceling my season tickets. So far I haven't done so because I really enjoy attending games with my family and friends. I justify my attendance in my own mind with the fact that at least those playing are adults who should have full awareness of the risks—and are paid a fortune to play.

One of the most devastating things that I see as a pediatric neurosurgeon living in an urban area in Texas, a state rife with firearms, is deadly or devastating injuries to the brain and spine from gun violence. I have unlimited sympathy for parents who live in economically depressed neighborhoods whose children are the innocent victims of drive-by shootings or gang violence. I struggle to understand the thought process of parents whose children's lives are ended or ruined because they own firearms that are not safely stored. I have taken care of children as young as four years of age who have encountered a gun in their home and shot themselves in the head by accident. I am currently caring for a fifteen-year-old girl whose father dropped his loaded firearm and discharged it accidentally. The bullet somehow went through a wall into the patient's room and struck his daughter in the head. After emergent surgery, she is alive but neurologically devastated. At the bedside, her father is stoic, but I can only imagine his guilt at every moment when he sees his daughter lying in bed without being able to talk or understand language. I have consulted on so many teenagers with known depression who commit suicide by accessing their parents' guns. Many of these suicide attempts are impulsive and would not have happened if a gun was not readily available at the very moment life's problems seemed insurmountable to those children. I recall taking care of a boy who ultimately died when he was shot in the head by his twin brother who thought he was playing with a toy. For these boys' parents, neglect in safely storing their guns ended the life of one of their sons and forever damaged the life of their surviving son who will have to live with the knowledge that he killed his brother.

In 2019, I coauthored a manuscript in the *Journal of Pediatric Surgery* in which we reviewed factors associated with gunshot wounds in children fifteen years of age or younger who were treated at our hospital, Children's Memorial Hermann Hospital, between 2001 and 2016.[5] During this period, 358 children were treated at Children's Memorial Hermann Hospital for gunshot wounds. We found that 45.5 percent of these incidents were intentional, 48.9 percent were accidental, and 4.7 percent were suicide attempts. A majority, 64 percent, occurred in a family residence. Guns were stored in a locked gun storage safe in only 1.7 percent of these cases, and we could only confirm that ammunition was stored separately from the gun in a single case. Only 4.2 percent of children who were injured by unsecured guns were placed in the custody of Child Protective Services (CPS). As a society, I know we can do better! Living in Texas, I understand the strong feelings that many law-abiding citizens have about guns, and I will not delve into the political debates about gun safety legislation. But safe storage is a position that should be supported by all. I will unequivocally state my opinion that there should be more education about safe gun storage and greater consequences for parents whose children are injured or killed when firearms are not safely stored.

Over the course of my career, I have witnessed so many complex situations that arise because there is such easy access to guns in our communities. I just recently saw a seventeen-year-old boy in my office who had sustained a severe traumatic brain injury several years ago. He had made a remarkable recovery overall, but injury to the frontal lobes of his brain had changed his personality and led to impulsive behavior. He had no real friends, had previously mentioned suicide, and had run away from home on several occasions. The boy's mother could not work because she was getting calls to pick her son up from the school so frequently due to behavioral issues. His father worried that his son would buy a gun legally when he turned eighteen but felt powerless to prevent him from doing so. As a police officer, he knew that the only way to prevent his son from legally purchasing a gun would be to have his legal adult rights rescinded. However, doing so required a higher burden of proving that his son was a danger to himself or others than was currently demonstrable. At the parents' request, I wrote a letter stating my opinion that this young man was a potential danger to himself and others and should not have access to a firearm, but it is unclear whether there will be sufficient evidence to prevent this when he becomes a legal adult very soon.

A rare but scary cause of traumatic brain injury I have seen a few times in my career is dog bites. The injuries I have seen and also read about in published reports have been in infants or very young children. Babies and young children are more likely to suffer skull fractures and brain injury from dog bites because of their short height, which makes their heads accessible to dogs.[6] Additionally, babies have large heads relative to their body size and thin skulls. The youngest baby I have ever cared for who had a devastating brain injury from a dog bite was only eight days old.

One particularly dramatic skull and brain injury from a dog bite that I managed occurred in an adorable eight-month-old boy named Kayden in 2013. Kayden was crawling on the floor when he was mauled by one of the three family dogs, an American bulldog. The dog had been around Kayden his whole life and had no history of aggressive behavior. His mom had briefly placed Kayden on the floor while the dog had been walking around the room, as she had done many times before. The dog attacked the baby without warning, biting the baby's head and causing

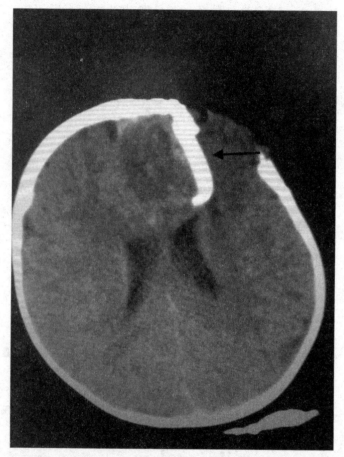

Figure 8. *Kayden's CT scan showing dramatic depressed skull fracture, marked by arrow, after a dog bite. The surrounding brain in the frontal lobe has been damaged and is a darker color than normal brain tissue.*

a severely depressed skull fracture and injury to the left frontal lobe of the brain.

Because of the obvious damage to the scalp and skull, with the baby's brain tissue actually visible at the bedside, a breathing tube was placed at the outside hospital where he was brought by his parents. Kayden was then transported by helicopter to our level one trauma center. I remember how distraught his parents were when I met them. Both of them were police officers, and Kayden's father actually worked in the canine unit (although the dog that caused the injury was a family dog not part of that unit). They are wonderful parents, both of whom have plenty of experience with dogs and never imagined that a terrible event like this could happen.

I took Kayden emergently to the operating room. In surgery, I debrided damaged brain in the left frontal lobe. Luckily, the brain that was damaged comes from an area of the frontal lobe that can often be removed without causing any impairment in neurological function. I elevated the depressed skull fracture and repaired it by drilling small holes in the loose bone and suturing it to normal adjacent bone. Then, I irrigated over and over again with fluid that contained antibiotic in it, as I was worried about the possibility of infection from a dog bite. My plastic surgery colleagues then did a beautiful job closing the badly damaged scalp.

Kayden made a complete recovery! Today, he is a completely normal eleven-year-old boy who is doing great in school and loves to play baseball. The only evidence of his injury is a scar that is largely hidden by hair. From time to time, his parents send me photos of Kayden along with most beautiful notes expressing their gratitude. The joy that these pictures and notes bring me cannot be put into words.

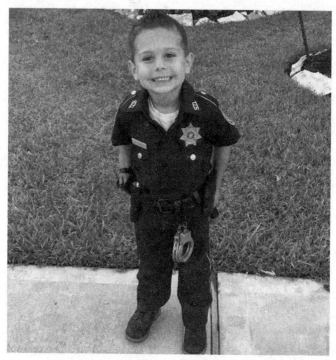

Figure 9. *Photo of Kayden at age four, taken three years after his dog bite. From his outfit, it appears that he is planning to follow in his parents' footsteps!*

Unfortunately, not all patients with traumatic brain injury experience happy endings. One of the most disturbing parts of my job is bearing witness to child abuse, which I, unfortunately, encounter quite frequently. There is nothing more heartbreaking than seeing a little baby who has been beaten or shaken with devastating effects to their brains or other body parts. It's simply hard to wrap your head around—how could anyone do this to an innocent baby? When my kids were babies, my wife and I certainly had our share of sleepless nights. I remember a few moments of frustration when our baby was crying inconsolably at 2:00 A.M. despite my trying everything I possibly could do to get her to go back to sleep. I tried changing her diaper, feeding her, rocking her, singing to her, and nothing worked. I remember thinking to myself, "Ah, now I get it. This is the moment where a young, frustrated, exhausted, uneducated parent might shake this child until she stops crying." Educating parents about the dangers of shaking their babies is a societal imperative. There is no remedy, of course, for the evil of caretakers who purposefully inflict harm on children. Seeing many victims of child abuse is demoralizing for the nurses, doctors, and social workers caring for these children in the hospital.

One of my least favorite situations as a pediatric neuro-surgeon is when I am asked to consult on whether a small bleed found on an imaging study in the subdural space (the space between the dura and the brain) was caused by child abuse. While subdural hemorrhages in babies and young children can be caused by abuse, they can also occur without abuse in some children either spontane-ously or after very minor trauma. When the brain bleed is associated with unexplained broken bones or other injuries, then there is no controversy. In some situations, it is simply hard to sort out whether abuse occurred. The worst thing, of course, is to send a child home to an unsafe situation. I have seen babies sent home from the hospital in equivocal circumstances who come back again with devastating injuries, or even die from subsequent abuse. On the other hand, the cruelty of removing a child from the custody of his or her parents if abuse did not occur cannot be overstated. I have seen situations in which children have been taken into CPS custody in which I am skeptical that the parents abused their child in any way. The parents' heartbreak is compounded by massive legal bills if they are even able to afford to hire an attorney to help them regain custody.

A career caring for children has forced me to bear witness over and over again to the devastation that can befall children after injuries to the brain or spine. I have seen both freak accidents and child abuse that wrecks the lives of children and their families. I have seen so many preventable injuries that I feel compelled to give unsolicited advice to parents about things like bicycle helmets, seat belts, and safe gun storage. I have witnessed the effects of societal ills such as gun violence and child abuse that leave me frustrated at the frequency of preventable tragedies in our society. Most of all, I come home from work every single day full of gratitude that my kids are safe and healthy. I sometimes hug them a little harder than I would have had I not seen something horrible at work that day. I never tell them why.

8

One Last Hope: Research Triumphs and Failures

Lisa and Brian struggled for years to have a successful pregnancy. After five miscarriages, their prayers were finally answered when Lisa gave birth to Luke at the age of forty. Luke would be their only child. Lisa and Brian were overjoyed, as they viewed Luke as their miracle baby.

At two months of age, Luke began having episodes in which he would briefly arch his back and then his eyes would look off to the side. His pediatrician thought that these episodes were from gastrointestinal (GI) reflux—a common problem in babies. When the episodes persisted, Luke was referred to a pediatric GI specialist, who agreed that Luke was having reflux and treated him with medication. The episodes persisted, and Luke was then sent to a pediatric neurologist who performed an electroencephalogram (EEG) to rule out seizures. The EEG did not detect any seizures. At age eleven months, on a Monday, Luke started vomiting and continued to do so for several days. At two visits to the pediatrician, on Tuesday and Friday, Luke's worried parents were told that Luke likely had a virus. By Sunday, Luke looked lethargic. Lisa and Brian decided to bring him to the emergency room at Miami Children's Hospital—later renamed Nicklaus Children's Hospital.

Brian drove to the hospital, and Lisa was in the back seat holding Luke. Suddenly, Lisa noticed that Luke's lips and face were turning blue. She shouted to Brian, who was an experienced nurse. Brian quickly pulled the car over and jumped into the back seat. Luke was clearly not breathing properly and Brian could not feel a pulse, so he began to perform CPR. Since they were less than a mile from the hospital, it was faster to drive the rest of the way rather than stop and call 911, so Lisa drove the last few blocks to the hospital, praying at the same time. When they arrived, Brian raced into the Emergency Department carrying Luke while simultaneously performing CPR. It was a dramatic scene.

When Luke arrived, the ED team sprang into action. They quickly put a breathing tube in, stabilized Luke—his pulse had thankfully returned—and took him for an emergent CT scan of the brain. The CT scan showed one of the largest brain tumors I had ever seen in the posterior fossa (the back portion of the brain that includes the cerebellum and brain stem). The tumor was blocking the circulation of CSF in the head, causing hydrocephalus, so I quickly placed a ventriculostomy—a drain to relieve the pressure. When the drain entered the ventricle, CSF streamed out under extremely high pressure. The next morning, we then sent Luke for an MRI scan to further characterize the tumor and then took him straight to the operating room to remove the tumor.

Removing a tumor of this size in a very small child has real hazards, but the surgery went perfectly. I was able to take out the entire tumor without complications. Lisa and Brian were so relieved—and then so distraught when the pathology came back. It was medulloblastoma, a malignant brain tumor. If Luke were older, the next step would have been radiation therapy, but the side effects of radiation to the brain can be devastating in babies, so it is typically deferred until the age of three. Instead, Luke would receive high dose chemotherapy followed by stem cell rescue. In other words, his little body would be blasted with drugs that would kill cancer cells, but were also powerful enough to destroy his normal bone marrow. Then, stem cells would hopefully "rescue" the bone marrow and enable production of healthy blood cells.

The drugs infused into Luke's body were given at such high doses that they caused tremendous damage to organs that had no cancer involvement whatsoever. He had repeated bouts of pneumonia, likely because chemotherapy had weakened his immune system. Several times, the pneumonia caused respiratory failure to the point that he required intubation (placement of a breathing tube). At age one, while intubated with respiratory failure, Luke additionally developed venous occlusive disease of the liver— the veins of his liver were damaged and became blocked, resulting in liver failure. Luke spent eight weeks in pediatric intensive care. For four of these weeks he required the breathing tube, and his survival was not certain. Somehow, he recovered and was eventually discharged from the hospital at eighteen months of age after completing chemotherapy.

Luke's developmental milestones were delayed because of all he had been through, but by age two he was walking, and things were looking up. At age five he enrolled in kindergarten! He was a happy and intelligent boy with no obvious problems other than high-frequency hearing loss from the prior chemotherapy. Lisa and Brian were thrilled. Unfortunately, at the age of five-and-a-half, Luke began having intermittent breathing problems that were initially diagnosed as repeated bouts of pneumonia. After months of evaluations, when these bouts worsened, he was again hospitalized and eventually had a lung biopsy that diagnosed end stage pulmonary fibrosis—his lungs had been irrevocably damaged by chemotherapy and had formed severe scar tissue that prevented them from functioning. Luke continued to worsen, and he was eventually put on the national lung transplant waiting list. Tragically, he deteriorated and died before a transplant could be performed.

From the day I removed Luke's brain tumor at eleven months of age until the day he died at age seven, his tumor never recurred. I tell Luke's story because he is one of several children I have cared for who died from the treatment—not the disease. Chemotherapy destroyed his liver and then his lungs—organs that had no cancer cells within them—and ultimately cost Luke his life. My own role in Luke's care was most prominent when he initially came to the hospital and I performed surgery, but I saw him many times thereafter and his parents became dear friends. I celebrated with them after every MRI following his surgery showed no tumor recurrence, and I saw their agony with each complication from chemotherapy. Luke's struggles and eventual death became a huge motivating factor for my research to find better and less toxic treatments for brain tumors in children. While seventeen years have passed since his dramatic arrival at Miami Children's Hospital, I still think of Luke quite often.

A major component of my career has been devoted to research trying to develop novel treatments for children like Luke. Parents like Lisa and Brian are desperate to try anything that can possibly save their child. I focus specifically on tumors in the posterior fossa, the region of the brain where Luke's tumor was found. Standard treatments for tumors like Luke's include surgical removal of the tumor, radiation therapy, and chemotherapy. None of these is a magic bullet, and all can cause major problems. Even after complete removal by surgery, malignant brain tumors often come back. Moreover, complications from brain tumor surgery in the posterior fossa, a challenging anatomical region of the brain, can cause permanent neurological problems. Radiation therapy can sometimes prevent tumors from recurring but is harmful to the developing nervous system. It can cause learning difficulties, hormonal problems, and sometimes even induce new malignant tumors. Chemotherapy can be effective against some brain tumors but not all. And while deaths like Luke's from chemotherapy are rare, significant side effects from chemotherapy are almost universal. When tumors come back despite surgery, radiation, and chemotherapy, alternative treatments have little chance of achieving a cure or long-term survival. The only thing left is clinical trials.

One day over twenty years ago, during my pediatric neurosurgery fellowship, we were operating on a child with a malignant brain tumor in the posterior fossa. We took out ninety-nine percent of the tumor, leaving behind a tiny bit that could not be safely removed because it was stuck to the brain stem. I knew what lay ahead for this four-year-old child—a difficult year of radiation therapy and chemotherapy and uncertain long-term survival. I thought to myself that, at this moment, the only known tumor in this child's body is this little bit stuck to the brain stem that I can see with my own eyes under the high-powered operating microscope. Yet, this child's whole body will soon be poisoned by drugs that affect many organs that have no tumor cells within them. The treatments will make her vomit frequently and will weaken her immune system. Her parents will agonize about so many toxic therapies given to their young daughter that cause discomfort that she is too young to understand. I asked several mentors why we don't infuse drugs directly into the brain to get high doses only where the tumor starts—and often comes back—while sparing the rest of the body? When I didn't receive good answers about why this hadn't been tried before, either from neurosurgical colleagues or from previously published journal articles, I decided to design experiments to test this new approach.

In the seven years that followed since I first had this idea, I performed numerous experiments in animals with promising results. These experiments proved that drugs could be administered directly into the fourth ventricle—the space in the posterior fossa where tumors often form and recur—without causing new neurological problems or any obvious damage to the brain. We could achieve extremely high drug levels locally in the brain while maintaining low drug levels in the blood stream. This result was exactly what we wanted—to blast the tumor cells while sparing the rest of the body. I hoped that in this way we could prevent tumors from coming back but avoid what happened to Luke—damage to organs that did not have tumors.

I was proud when my experiments led to the first clinical trial testing this treatment approach in humans. There are so many great ideas tested in laboratories, but only a small percentage of these ideas go "from bench to bedside," leading to new treatments for patients. In our first pilot clinical trial, which began in Houston in 2013, we infused methotrexate—a drug often used intravenously to treat some brain tumors and other cancers—into the back of the brain in children who had failed other treatments. I was overwhelmed with delight when there was shrinkage of the tumor in all three patients we enrolled with medulloblastoma, the most common malignant brain tumor in children (still a very rare disease). Two additionally enrolled patients had a different type of tumor—ependymoma. One of these patients failed our trial, with the tumor growing back quickly despite the infusions. The other patient's tumor initially seemed to respond to treatment, but eventually his tumor grew back, too. I knew that I needed a new clinical trial testing infusion of a different drug into the fourth ventricle that would hopefully more effectively treat ependymoma.

Jocelyn was the first patient enrolled in my next clinical trial. My trial was likely her last chance to try to conquer a foe that to date had been unconquerable—the horrible cancer in the back of her brain. Jocelyn had her first brain tumor surgery when she was only six months old. Her parents noticed that she was tilting her head to the side, and she began intermittently vomiting. When the vomiting worsened, a CT scan of the brain was performed. It showed a large tumor located in the posterior fossa—the same area of the brain as Luke's tumor. Surgery in her hometown, San Antonio, Texas, revealed the unfortunate diagnosis of anaplastic ependymoma, a relentless cancer that often comes back over and over again. She received chemotherapy, but the tumor came roaring back despite the grueling treatments endured by her little body. She underwent her second surgery at the age of two. At this second operation, her neurosurgeon encountered a tumor that could not be completely removed safely because it was stuck to nerves that control the ability to swallow. Shortly after this second surgery, she underwent radiation therapy in the hope that it would kill the tumor cells that had been left behind. Unfortunately, the tumor again recurred, and she underwent her third surgery at the age of four to remove as much tumor as possible once again. This was followed by more radiation therapy—this time "gamma knife" radiosurgery, in which a high dose of radiation is given in a single session. Less than a year later, the tumor was back yet again. Jocelyn then underwent her fourth surgical resection followed by a clinical trial in Dallas testing another chemotherapy drug. When this trial failed and the tumor again recurred, her parents came to Houston to enroll in our clinical trial for recurrent ependymoma. With no proven treatments left to offer, our clinical trial was likely her last shot at survival.

Jocelyn enrolled in my brand-new clinical trial testing infusions into the back of the brain of a drug called 5-azacytidine, which had shown promising activity in the laboratory against her specific tumor type. I remember meeting Jocelyn's parents, Nicole and Michael, for the first time. They are a wonderful couple who had struggled through so much hardship with their adorable first child. Nicole and Michael were realistic about Jocelyn's prognosis, but they clung to the small hope that a cure could be found. They wanted to leave no stone unturned in their attempts to save their beloved little girl. I thought to myself how cruel it was for this couple to have suffered so much. So often, the worst tragedies seem to happen to the nicest people. I was so hopeful that the new treatment we were trying, for the first time in humans, would be the answer to their prayers.

It was clear to me that Jocelyn's prior surgeries and treatments had taken a large toll on her small six-year-old body. She had hearing loss on the right side, and her smile was crooked because the tumor and/or her prior surgeries had affected her facial nerve, which lies in the space occupied by her tumor. When she walked, she was slightly unsteady, but she loved to skip. Each time I examined Jocelyn, I asked her to walk so I could assess the steadiness of her gait. Instead of walking, she always skipped, going above and beyond what I had asked for. It was literally the cutest thing. I became increasingly attached to this adorable little girl skipping down the hall who had been dealt such an unfair fate. I desperately hoped that my investigational treatment would help her.

On February 1, 2017, I performed Jocelyn's fifth brain surgery. I removed the majority of her tumor, leaving behind a small amount that could not be safely removed. I then placed a catheter in the tumor bed and attached the catheter to a reservoir that was implanted underneath her skin. Through this reservoir, via a small needle inserted into the skin, we would infuse the 5-azacytidine right where the small bits of tumor were left behind in the back of Jocelyn's brain. Over the next two months, Jocelyn received weekly infusions through the reservoir. Each infusion required great effort on the part of Jocelyn's parents—a three-hour drive in each direction back and forth from San Antonio. Every week I examined her before and after these infusions, and I was encouraged that she looked and felt great. With each examination, I assessed her walking, and I always smiled as she skipped down the hall. I silently prayed that the infusions were working.

The moment of truth came sooner than I wanted. Fluid that we sampled from the reservoir appeared to be infected, so I decided to order an MRI scan right away. We had planned an MRI scan after twelve infusions, and she had only received eight, but the infection required removal of the reservoir. An MRI scan would reveal information not only about the infection but would also tell us whether the treatments had worked.

I remember to this day sitting in my office while Jocelyn was in the MRI scanner. Every two minutes I kept hitting refresh on the computer screen. I was so anxious, and I could not focus on anything else. When the images finally came up on my computer, I slumped into my chair, devastated. The MRI not only showed evidence of infection around the reservoir, but the tumor had massively progressed in spite of the infusions. I felt as though her tumor was cruelly laughing at me and my attempts to stop its growth.

I knew what came next—the horrible task of sharing the MRI findings with Jocelyn's parents. I reluctantly got up from my desk and began to walk to the hospital wards. I usually walk briskly from place to place, as I am always in a rush, but this time I walked slowly. I tried to make myself strong, but I felt weak and fragile and slightly sick to my stomach. The minute Jocelyn's parents saw my face, they knew that the news was not good. We walked together to a private area, and I pulled up the MRI scan to show them. As I began to talk, I was overcome by emotion. At that time, my own youngest child was the same age as Jocelyn, six years old, and I thought about how I would feel if I were receiving this news about him. I also thought about how filled with life Jocelyn was when she skipped down the hall. I couldn't get that image out of my mind. As my words came out describing the MRI scan, I began to cry uncontrollably. Other times in my career I had felt tears in my eyes while talking to a family and held them back, but I had never cried like this in front of a patient. It was almost as though I was releasing emotions bottled up from years of seeing many beautiful children die of these unrelenting tumors.

Years later, I asked Jocelyn's parents if they remembered my crying during this conversation and how this made them feel. I was worried that my lack of control over my emotions had been unprofessional. After all, my own pain obviously paled in comparison to that of Jocelyn's parents, and my job was to comfort them. I was relieved when Jocelyn's dad recalled that my tears during this conversation made him and Jocelyn's mom feel as though I was truly in it with them, and they expressed their gratitude for this. They also told me that despite the fact that the treatment had failed, they had no regrets about enrolling in the clinical trial. Jocelyn died of her tumor two months later, on June 8, 2017. From time to time, when I am treating other patients with the same disease, an image of her skipping down the hall enters my mind, and a sad half-smile comes across my face.

Although I have not yet cured a child with a recurrent brain cancer, I have had surprisingly promising results in some patients. One such patient I will never forget is Jordan, an amazing nineteen-year-old boy from Alabama who was the first patient enrolled in my very first pilot clinical trial. He would be the first human being ever to receive chemotherapy directly into the fourth ventricle of the brain. In 2004, Jordan was diagnosed with medulloblastoma. After surgery, he underwent radiation therapy and chemotherapy. His family was so hopeful when his MRI scans were clean for five years. Cruelly, his tumor then recurred, and three additional chemotherapy drugs failed to keep his tumor from growing.

When I met Jordan, I was struck by his charisma and his poise. He understood the horrible situation he was in, as standard treatments for recurrent medulloblastoma rarely work. He probably had around three months to live. Here was a sweet kid who deserved to have his whole life in front of him who was being told that that his time on Earth would be counted in months, not years. And yet, he was calm and at peace, strengthened by his deep Christian faith. He had large areas of recurrent tumor in multiple spots in the brain and also coating the spine. As a result of the tumor in the brain, his walking was unsteady and he had double vision and nystagmus—jerking of the eyes back and forth. He wore thick prism glasses to improve his double vision.

When I spoke to Jordan about enrolling in the trial, he asked me about being the very first person to participate in this experimental treatment. I told him, "Young man, there always has to be that brave first person." Jordan's mom, Kathy, later told me that at that moment, she thought to herself that if I was looking for a brave young man, I had found the right guy.

Jordan underwent surgery to implant a catheter and reservoir in the fourth ventricle. We removed very little tumor because there was so much tumor all over his brain that it did not make sense to perform aggressive surgery. After he recovered from surgery, we gave eighteen infusions of the chemotherapy drug methotrexate into his fourth ventricle. His family and I felt that our prayers had been answered when his tumor was smaller on his follow-up MRI three months after his first infusion. I thought that this pilot clinical trial was more likely to show safety than efficacy, but the treatment was actually working! We gave another eighteen infusions over the next three months, and Jordan's next MRI looked even better. We wound up giving Jordan seventy-two infusions over the course of a year.

That first year was, in many ways, a wonderful year for Jordan and his family. He had no side effects from the infusions, and each week his walking improved to the point where he could exercise alone on a treadmill. His double vision improved to the point where he no longer had to wear the special prism glasses made for him by his eye doctor. His nystagmus—the spontaneous jerking of his eyes—also improved dramatically. He felt well enough to return to Costa Rica, where he had previously been involved in a missionary training program. He also went on a Christian mission trip to the Dominican Republic, and this trip was so meaningful to Jordan. I felt an immense sense of triumph when the treatment I had designed seemed to be working so well and devastation when it ultimately failed. Unfortunately, one of his tumors regrew at the end of the first year of infusions, so we took

Jordan out of our protocol. Despite other attempted treatments, Jordan tragically died of progressive tumor a year later—over two years after I first met him when he had been told that his life expectancy was three months.

I become very close to so many of my patients and their families, but I certainly have a special bond with the kids enrolled in my research trials and their families. It is hard to put into words how emotionally invested I am in these kids. When our infusions make tumors shrink, I share tears of joy with their parents. When tumors grow despite treatment, the impact on me is immense—and I know that the pain I am feeling is nothing compared to the agony of the child's parents, grandparents, siblings, and other loved ones. Although I have not yet achieved a cure, I am not even close to giving up this fight. The memories of Luke and Jocelyn and Jordan and so many other children push me to do my very best to find better treatments for these relentless tumors.

As medical students and residents carve out their unique career paths, many shy away from research. Some simply have a greater passion for clinical medicine. Some might be inclined to include research as a component of their career, but they are intimidated by others whom they perceive as smarter or better equipped to answer scientific questions than they are. So many students and residents are advised that they can be great clinicians or great scientists, but it's impossible to excel at both. Scientific experiments, they are told, are best performed by PhD scientists who are better trained in scientific methods and can spend their days designing and performing experiments while clinicians have so much of their time occupied by clinics and/or surgeries.

I have an alternative perspective. At no point in my life—not in high school, college, medical school, residency, nor as an attending neurosurgeon—have I ever been the smartest person in the room. Furthermore, I certainly have had relatively little scientific training compared to many people in academic medicine. I was a history major in college, and the only science courses I took were the basic premedical requirements. The first time I ever worked in a laboratory was during the summer between my first and second years in medical school. I spent that summer working in an infectious disease laboratory and quickly figured out that basic science experiments were not for me. The biggest reason for this is that I never thought I had sufficient skills, training, or intelligence to come up with a meaningful scientific experiment that had not already been performed by someone else. After deciding to become a neurosurgeon, I spent four months at the end of my third year of medical school working in a brain tumor laboratory. In this laboratory, neurosurgeons performed animal surgeries testing delivery of drugs into the brain to treat malignant brain tumors, and this was right up my alley. I saw that clinicians could form ideas based upon observations from clinical encounters with patients and then test those ideas in the laboratory—with the goal of creating better treatments for diseases they saw every day. However, I still had doubts about my ability to think of original research projects and design my own experiments.

In residency, we had a mandatory research year, and I worked on another translational research project involving direct drug delivery into the brain. Under the direction of my pediatric neurosurgery mentor, Dr. Souweidane, I performed experiments in rodents testing drug delivery into the brain stem to treat incurable tumors that occur in this region of the brain. Dr. Souweidane is a clinical neurosurgeon—without a PhD—whose scientific ideas are driven by the devastating conditions he treats in children. During that year, under Dr. Souweidane's supervision, I learned how to ask a scientific question and design an experiment to answer that question. I learned how to write a proposal, gather the appropriate resources, perform experiments, and report my findings in oral presentations at national meetings and in published manuscripts.

Like Dr. Souweidane, my research originated from an idea that came directly from my clinical practice. I am living proof that scientific contributions can be made by clinicians who do not have a PhD or even a strong scientific background. There is a role for scientific discovery inspired by clinical observations to which only clinicians have access. I have been humbled over and over again, as I have still not cured a single child with a recurrent malignant tumor. There are too many kids like Jocelyn and Jordan whose tumors have progressed despite my clinical trials (and trials at other institutions that were tried before or after mine). But I do not underestimate the importance of the hope and possibly extended time that clinical trials provide to families whose children have failed all standard treatments. Many of these families have been told at their local hospitals that all treatments that have a chance of working have already failed, and that hospice or palliative care is the next logical step. But the power of hope is so great that these families search throughout the world for clinical trials and travel for experimental treatments, often at great personal expense. Tragically, I have seen families sell their homes to raise funds to participate in clinical trials that only have a small chance of saving their child's life. The dedication of these families never ceases to amaze me. It has been an incredibly meaningful part of my career to at least try to come up with new treatments rather than simply accept that dismal outcomes are inevitable for these precious children. Although I always provide an honest assessment to my patients and their families when the odds are stacked against them, their indomitable spirit lifts me up and pushes me to do my very best.

9

Exhilaration and Despair: Pediatric Neurosurgery in Low- and Middle-Income Countries

As our van pulled into the makeshift clinic at Hospital Bernard Mevs in Port-au-Prince, Haiti, the first thing that struck me was the huge crowd of parents and babies awaiting our team's arrival. As I stepped out of the van, I was astonished to see that many of these babies had the largest heads I had ever seen—literally as big as watermelons. Some of these heads were more than twice the size of a normal baby's head. They were attached to little bodies, many of which were emaciated from malnourishment. These babies had severe untreated hydrocephalus—a condition in which the fluid produced continuously by the brain is not absorbed properly. When hydrocephalus occurs, the fluid spaces in the brain (called the ventricles) get bigger and bigger and cause the head to enlarge rapidly. Meanwhile, normal brain tissue becomes damaged by pressure resulting from the fluid build-up. While hydrocephalus is seen in all countries throughout the world, only in low- and middle-income countries would a child have a head this large from not receiving timely care. I had treated many children with hydrocephalus in the United States, as hydrocephalus is the most common condition treated by pediatric neurosurgeons, but I had never seen babies who looked like this. Images of these huge heads attached to tiny bodies were indelibly burned into my brain.

After learning that a team of pediatric neurosurgeons would be coming to Port-au-Prince, the parents of these children traveled from all over the country, some of them for days, in the desperate hope that their babies could be treated. The families waited patiently outside in the intense heat for many hours. The lucky ones had chairs, but there were not enough chairs for everyone, so most were sprawled out on the hot concrete pavement. These families endured this hardship because it was literally the only chance for their babies to receive the operations they needed. There were four neurosurgeons in the whole country of Haiti at the time, and none had any specific pediatric neurosurgery training. None of them routinely took care of children with hydrocephalus—particularly poor children whose parents could not pay for medical treatments.

As we prepared to start evaluating the patients, I quickly estimated that there were approximately eighty children waiting to be evaluated. I had a sinking feeling in my stomach, as I knew that we only had enough time and equipment to perform twenty-five surgeries. This meant that most of these families would be turned away without treatment, and many of these babies would eventually die.

I had the unenviable task of deciding who would live and who would die. I thought to myself, who am I to make these decisions? What right do I have to "play God?" While these thoughts never completely left my mind—and still haven't years later—I had no choice but to try to set them aside and focus on helping as many kids as I could. I chose the twenty-five children with the best chance of having a good surgical outcome and becoming functional adults one day. After seeing each patient, I put each one's crude hospital chart in one of three piles—no, yes, and maybe. The "no" pile included older kids with enormous heads whose CT scans showed massive amounts of fluid and little brain tissue. These children's hydrocephalus had gone on for so long that their brain tissue was thinned out and damaged beyond any reasonable possibility of repair. The "no" pile also included babies who appeared too malnourished to safely undergo surgery, or babies with high fevers—mostly from respiratory illnesses and some from malaria—which rendered surgery unsafe. I thought to myself how tragically unlucky these babies were who happened to have fevers at that moment in time. By the time the next surgical team arrived a few months later, their heads would be dramatically larger and their brains irrevocably damaged, and they would likely end up in the "no" pile once more. Like me, our team's anesthesiologists also had the unenviable task of playing God. Back home, an elective surgery could be delayed for a few weeks for a child with a common cold. Here, our anesthesiologists knew that if a surgery was prevented by a cold, it would likely never happen. But the elevated risks of anesthesia and the lack of adequate resources to care for a sick child postoperatively forced our team to err on the side of not performing surgeries in kids who had fevers or were coughing or sneezing. It was a horrible feeling for every member of our team.

The "yes" pile included the youngest babies who had the most brain tissue to save and otherwise appeared healthy. The "maybe" pile included patients who were not quite as likely to have good outcomes as those in the "yes" pile but were decent surgical candidates. In truth, the "maybe" pile was essentially a waiting list; these children would possibly receive surgery, but only if there weren't too many better candidates. Typically, around half of the patients in the "maybe" pile ultimately made it to the "yes" pile. After seeing all eighty kids in the clinic, and after eliminating from consideration those patients vetoed by our anesthesiologists, our team looked over the patients' charts and imaging studies one more time. I then made the final decision regarding which twenty-five patients would make it onto our surgical schedule. With the help of a Creole translator, we informed parents on the "no" list that we would not be able to help their babies. There were a few tears, but most of the parents reacted quite stoically, without even a change in facial expression. It was almost as if these parents were so used to suffering that they had come to expect it. I knew how badly they must have been hurting inside after traveling for days in the hope of their babies being saved only to be told that it wasn't possible. I felt powerless and guilty. I thought to myself how lucky I am—through no merit whatsoever—to have been born into my parents' home in Miami, Florida, instead of a place like this. And how lucky my own children are, as they are no more worthy than these children in Haiti of receiving appropriate medical care.

Trying to help children with neurosurgical conditions in low- and middle-income countries has been one of the greatest passions of my career. The roots of this passion lie in the values instilled in me by my parents, both of whom are very focused on public service. As I mentioned in chapter two, my first experiences with neurosurgery abroad were accompanying my father on three ophthalmology medical missions in high school and college. Many years later, when I had gained the skills in my own profession to actually make a difference, I was determined to make global pediatric neurosurgery an important part of my career.

My first experience with international neurosurgery came earlier than expected. Dr. Neil Feldstein, a pediatric neurosurgeon from Columbia University in New York City, came across town one day to give a lecture to our program. Dr. Feldstein described a recent pediatric neurosurgery medical mission he had led to Guatemala. His team had performed about twenty surgeries on children who otherwise would not have received timely care—or perhaps any care at all—for various neurosurgical problems. I was overcome by excitement, as one of my doubts about becoming a neurosurgeon had been whether I could incorporate treating the underserved. After the lecture, I literally begged Dr. Feldstein to consider taking me on his next trip. I think that Dr. Feldstein appreciated my passion for this project, and he agreed to do so.

I wound up accompanying Dr. Feldstein twice to Guatemala, first in 1999, as a second-year resident, and then in 2001, as a fourth-year resident. These trips were incredible experiences. From a learning standpoint, I was exposed to cases that are much rarer in the United States than in Guatemala. In particular, I participated in more surgeries for closed neural tube defects during my two trips to Guatemala than during the rest of my residency combined. Closed neural tube defects are congenital conditions in which the bones of the spinal column do not form completely. The underlying spinal cord is often tethered to fat or other structures and must be detached to function optimally. Assisting in these surgeries provided me with an operative experience for tethered spinal cords that surpassed any available experience in the United States. Most important, participating in these trips showed me that it was actually possible within the field of neurosurgery to treat underserved patients abroad.

Over the course of my career, I have organized or participated in over twenty international humanitarian pediatric neurosurgical missions, including visits to Honduras, Guatemala, Peru, Uganda, Mexico, and Haiti. In these countries and in many others, poor children often receive inadequate or delayed treatment or no treatment at all, which amounts to a death sentence for many of them. It's a lesson I first learned on that trip to Honduras when I met Marcela—whose story I told in chapter four—but have been reminded of many times since. The world can be unfair, and the fate of children can rest on nothing more than chance. Marcela is only alive today because she had the good fortune to be admitted to Hospital Escuela during my visit, and so many pieces fell into place that could have just as easily not worked out. Bringing Marcela to New York saved her life, but this is not a model that can be replicated on a large scale for the many other deserving children at Hospital Escuela or elsewhere.

There have been a few other children since Marcela whom I have brought to the United States over the years, but the sad fact remains that it is financially and logistically impossible to bring even a tiny percentage of sick children from low- or middle-income countries to a more developed country for care. An alternative approach is to try to perform as many operations as possible on children in their home countries during medical missions. But even performing twenty or twenty-five surgeries on each of these trips feels like a drop in the bucket. It is life-changing for some but still excludes so many others. Choosing who will have surgery and survive and who will not have surgery and die is a truly horrible feeling. Additionally, follow-up care after visiting surgeons leave town is often inadequate or nonexistent. This is particularly problematic if complications arise. Perhaps most important, operating on a small cohort of patients in another country helps those patients, but does nothing to change the system in that country for the better. Patients in the general population cannot rely for care on foreign surgeons who show up sporadically and then return to their home countries.

A much better means of achieving lasting change is to help train local neurosurgeons from low- and middle-income countries to perform the best possible surgeries for the children under their care. This is the "teach a man to fish" concept from the old adage, "Give a man a fish, and you feed him for a day; teach a man to fish and you feed him for a lifetime." There are two ways of doing this, both with advantages and disadvantages. The first way is to bring neurosurgeons from their home countries to the United States or another highly developed country for training. Doing so is an extraordinary opportunity for these neurosurgeons to learn from masters in the field and to dream big about what could be accomplished in their home countries. Unfortunately, due to medical malpractice insurance issues, many visiting neurosurgeons are only permitted to observe surgery rather than participate, which is less impactful. Also unfortunately, many visiting surgeons from low- and middle-income countries decide to try to stay in the United States after training rather than returning to their home countries afterward. Who can blame them, as they quickly see that surgeons here have more advanced equipment, more support from their hospitals, and dramatically better lifestyles than their colleagues back home? But there is a huge shortage of surgical subspecialists in most low- and middle-income countries, and it is tragic, in my opinion, to lose the opportunity to have these surgeons return to their communities where they could potentially make a bigger difference.

The second way of accomplishing the "teach a man to fish" concept is to train neurosurgeons in their own environments using the resources and technology they have at hand. In an effort to have the greatest impact on the largest number of patients, my work in low- and middle-income countries has evolved over time. Early in my career, I went with a team of physicians, nurses, and volunteers and performed as many surgeries as possible with limited interaction with local physicians. Now, when I travel on one of these medical mission trips, I still perform surgery, but I am mainly focused on training local neurosurgeons who perform the surgeries under my supervision. In this way, I hope to do the most good for the most children on a long-term basis in these countries. I work toward the day when children no longer need to wait for the arrival of foreign doctors in the hopes of being one of the lucky few who are treated by a visiting neurosurgeon.

For example, a large focus of my time in Haiti has been working with Dr. Yudy Lafortune at Hospital Bernard Mevs in the capital, Port-au-Prince. Dr. Lafortune was the first fellow in Project Medishare's neurosurgery fellowship program. I have traveled to Haiti ten times, and I have worked with Dr. Lafortune on many of these trips. It has been incredibly rewarding to observe the tremendous progression in Dr. Lafortune's surgical skills over time. Led by Dr. John Ragheb, director of pediatric neurosurgery at Nicklaus Children's Hospital in Miami, a series of visiting pediatric neurosurgeons have spent time training Dr. Lafortune in his own environment in Port-au-Prince. When these efforts first started, Dr. Lafortune had little familiarity with modern surgical techniques to treat the most common pediatric neurosurgical conditions. Now, he is fully capable of taking great care of children with these conditions. Dr. Lafortune is the only neurosurgeon in Haiti who is trained to perform modern endoscopic neurosurgical operations—minimally invasive surgeries performed with a small camera via a small incision—to treat hydrocephalus. Most important, Dr. Lafortune has maintained a tremendous work ethic, working day and night to provide the best care he can for every child. He is respectful of every family, no matter what financial circumstances they have, and is always willing to take the time to explain things to the parents of his patients.

Unfortunately, not all the doctors in the countries I have visited are as caring as Dr. Lafortune. I have witnessed some who display a stunning indifference to the suffering of the poor children in their care, while lavishing time and attention on the children of wealthy families. I vividly recall making rounds one day with a neurosurgeon in a low-income country. We first made rounds at a public hospital that was overflowing with extremely sick children who were at risk of dying from brain tumors, hydrocephalus, infections, and many other disastrous situations. This neurosurgeon spent less than a minute with each patient and didn't answer the questions of a single parent. Later that same day, he took me to his private practice where he saw a single patient who came to his office for evaluation of headaches. The child had a normal MRI of the brain and did not need any neurosurgical intervention. But because he came from a wealthy family and the patient's parents were paying cash for the consultation, the neurosurgeon spent over an hour examining the child and answering the parents' many questions. The entire time, I was thinking about all of the poor children at the public hospital with real and desperate neurosurgical problems that he had completely ignored earlier the same day. I vowed to myself never to work again with this particular neurosurgeon.

Citizens and politicians in the United States and other developed nations often debate the merits of varying approaches to healthcare, but it is hard to overstate the difference in care between the developed and developing world—especially for poor children. In some of the countries I have visited in Central America and Africa, the healthcare system is so grossly inadequate that even easily cured diseases often go untreated, resulting in unnecessary severe disability or death. A common pattern of employment is that physicians work at public hospitals that serve indigent patients in the mornings. They earn tiny salaries for this work from the government. These salaries are completely inadequate to cover even basic living expenses for themselves and their families. The public hospitals are teeming with patients who desperately need care, but the physicians cannot work there full-time because they need to have supplemental income to provide for their families. In addition, there are not enough operating rooms or appropriate equipment at the public hospitals. Something is always broken, and this can lead to indifference by some staff members. I have seen patients die because the elevator is broken, and the patient cannot be transported from the emergency room on the ground floor to the operating room on a higher floor for emergency surgery.

These physicians earn the majority of their income by going to private practices in the afternoons. There they see the small minority who can afford to pay cash for private care. They see relatively few patients and perform surgeries as needed on these patients in smaller private hospitals. I feel so lucky that I am a salaried employee with no financial incentive to treat patients differently based upon their social status or ability to pay. Whether a patient comes from a wealthy family with private insurance or is indigent and has no health insurance, I perform the exact same surgery and give the patient and family the exact same time and attention. Most of the time, I don't even know the insurance status of my patients. In reality, only a tiny percentage of physicians around the world are lucky enough to practice medicine in a situation like mine without any perverse financial incentives, a truly sad state for our world.

The vast majority of neurosurgeons I have encountered in my travels are amazing human beings who desperately want to do the very best they can to help each patient. Many of them are frustrated by the limited equipment available to them and the inadequate health care systems in which they work. I have told many of them, with great sincerity, that I am jealous of them. Why would I be jealous of them, some ask, considering the great resources at my disposal? My answer is that they have an opportunity that I wish I had—to change pediatric neurosurgery in their countries in a profound way. There are plenty of excellent pediatric neurosurgeons in Houston and every other major city in the United States. If I am not available, my patients can get great care from one of my partners or from neurosurgeons at another center in our city or one nearby. But if a neurosurgeon in a low- or middle-income country learns a new technique that is not currently offered locally, he or she can permanently change care in his or her community and country for the better—and also pass along their newly gained skills to their own trainees.

One example of a neurosurgeon who has done exactly this is Dr. Tulio Murillo, the neurosurgeon I mentioned in chapter four who emergently placed Marcela's shunt. I met Dr. Murillo during my first trip to Honduras. At the time, he and I were both senior residents. Dr. Murillo is one of the most incredible human beings and neurosurgeons with whom I have had the honor of working. He lived and breathed neurosurgery, reading every neurosurgery article and textbook he could get his hands on to better his knowledge. He was in the hospital day and night, saving lives with tremendous skill and compassion. After he finished his training at Hospital Escuela in Tegucigalpa, he traveled to the United States for fellowship training in endovascular neurosurgery, a modern neurosurgical sub-specialty in which problems like brain aneurysms—blisters on arteries of the brain that can rupture and bleed—can be treated in a minimally invasive manner by advancing catheters through a groin puncture into the brain. Dr. Murillo then returned to Honduras, where he was the first in his country to perform these procedures. He has saved countless lives and singlehandedly advanced neurosurgical care in his country.

My involvement in global neurosurgery has provided some of the most rewarding experiences of my life and career. Performing surgeries and teaching neurosurgeons in low- and middle-income countries, I am able to help children who otherwise face preventable death or severe disability. These experiences are extremely gratifying, in part, because they are pure medicine—free of the interference of insurance companies or other annoying bureaucratic barriers I face at home. On the other hand, my experiences abroad always make me appreciate the amazing technology and resources available to me when I care for patients at home. I have learned that I can operate effectively with far fewer instruments than I have at home. I have had to finish operations in a dark operating room with only a headlight when the electricity in the hospital has gone out. When I get back home, I am less likely to complain about a pair of microscissors that isn't sharp enough, or other such minor things. I am just grateful for what I have.

Even with the progress I have witnessed in places like Honduras or Haiti, I never lose sight of the enormous disparities that exist in the world. I often think about the other sick children in the pediatric ward of Hospital Escuela—the children who were not as lucky as Marcela. I also think of the Haitian babies in the "no" pile who are all now either dead or severely disabled but could have lived if they had undergone a timely surgery that only takes an hour to perform. I look forward, in my lifetime, to seeing incremental progress in global neurosurgery that will hopefully decrease the tremendous inequity between the care available in developed and less developed countries.

Epilogue

As I reflect on my career as a pediatric neurosurgeon, I am filled with gratitude that I have had the opportunity to spend my life doing something so profoundly meaningful. I feel so incredibly lucky that each day I get to pour my heart into saving the lives of children. I have been lifted up to the greatest heights when I have succeeded in this endeavor. I also have been deeply humbled by the limitations of my work and have shared the most devastating lows with families whose children I have been unable to save.

As this journey has progressed over the past quarter of a century, I am also grateful for all I have learned and how much I have grown. I have endured the stress that accompanies having a job that doesn't pause on nights, weekends, or holidays, and frequently being pulled in many directions at once. I have wrestled with the uncertainty of surgical outcomes involving the brain and spine and have learned to face—while never fully accepting—the rare but horrible circumstance of a child being worse after surgery than they were beforehand. I often joke with parents of children for whom I have cared over a period of many years that some of the increasingly gray hair on my head comes from all that we have been through together.

Experiences abroad have truly opened my eyes to the inequities in our world and to how fortunate I am in countless ways. While I witness innumerable tragedies caring for children with devastating diseases in the United States, working in low- and middle-income countries is often the most profound reminder of how drastically societal inequality affects children with illness, who are often the most vulnerable members of society. My life has been deeply enriched by witnessing the heart of families in underserved countries who—without resentment—fight for their children when the system is indifferent or even outright hostile to them.

When I chose to become a pediatric neurosurgeon, my decision stemmed from a fascination with the brain and all of its mystery and the excitement of performing complex surgeries on this powerful, defining organ. But as the years go by, I am most amazed by the power of the heart—not the physical heart that pumps blood throughout our bodies but the heart in a figurative sense as the center of our emotions. When taking care of precious children who might die or have bad outcomes, every member of our team has to put his or her heart on the line. Our nurses, residents, scrub techs, and colleagues make themselves vulnerable, knowing that our best efforts may be inadequate. My patients and their families further amaze me with their hearts as they fight so hard with tremendous optimism, grit, and stamina to overcome heartbreaking diseases that they don't deserve ever to have faced. The children with brain tumors who participate in clinical trials and their extraordinary families blow me away with their hearts and their hope as they fight for their lives against the odds.

I hope that the stories I have shared about the amazing children and families I have encountered in my journey have touched your heart in some way. The greatest reward for me would be to learn that these stories have influenced others to support children and their families who are fighting to overcome devastating diseases—or to do anything they can, big or small, to help someone else in need.

Acknowledgments

I am incredibly grateful to so many people who have helped me tremendously in my career and with this book. First and foremost, I want to thank my amazing patients and their wonderful families. There are not enough words to thank the parents of my patients for entrusting me with the care of their beloved children and for their limitless love and kindness to me. Thank you—to both my patients and your families—for inspiring me with your courage in the face of the unthinkable and for bringing so much meaning to my life. I want to convey special thanks to five patients who are featured prominently in this book and their parents who permitted me to share their stories: Kayden Chapa and his parents Sandi and Alex, Jocelyn Diaz (deceased) and her parents Nicole and Michael Diaz, Jordan Grisham (deceased) and his parents Kathy and Daryl Grisham, Garrett Heble and his parents Holly and Kurt, Marcela Lainez Oseguera and her parents Aracely and Juan Carlos, and Luke Sturgill (deceased) and his parents Lisa and Brian. Each of these patients and families touched my heart in a truly special way and helped to alter my path as a neurosurgeon and human being. There are many other patients and their families not listed here whose stories are told under pseudonyms or not told in this book about whom I could say the same thing.

I would like to express my heartfelt gratitude to Jessica Case and Claiborne Hancock, the amazing team at Pegasus Books. Thank you for taking a chance on a first-time author! Thank you for your encouragement, your insightful editing and for guiding me through all aspects of the publication process. I will always be grateful to both of you. I am so grateful to Meghan Jusczak, who did an amazing job publicizing the book. Libby Duke and Sydney Burger of Thrive Global additionally went above and beyond to publicize the book. Additional thanks to Maria Fernandez for her help with interior design and production, Faceout Studio for their help with the book cover, Drew Wheeler for help with copy editing, and Daniel O'Connor for proofreading. Additional thanks to Samantha Lombardo for her amazing help with logistics for the book and so many other aspects of my life.

I would also like to thank my colleagues, family members, and friends who read drafts or chapters of *Brain and Heart* and gave me encouragement and critical feedback. David Martin is an extremely talented writer who helped me compose the proposal for *Brain and Heart* and helped me formulate chapter 1. Kim Schefler, my publishing attorney and agent, provided great advice and guidance throughout the publishing process. I was so honored that Arianna Huffington wrote the most generous foreword for the book. Brad Meltzer went above and beyond in reading the proposal and selected chapters and sharing the wisdom he has gained from his vast writing and publishing experience. Adam Grant, Allyson Lack, Emilie Martinez, Ken Richman, Manish Shah, and Jay Wellons read either the proposal or selected chapters and gave me both advice and encouragement.

My single most important editor was my wife, Amy Schefler, who helped me formulate ideas and read every draft of every chapter numerous times. Other immediate family members who spent a great deal of time reading chapters and providing thoughtful critiques were my parents, Adele and Joel Sandberg, my sisters, Sheryl and Michelle Sandberg, my brothers-in-law, Marc Bodnick, Tom Bernthal, and Ken Schefler, and my children, Dalia and Benjamin Sandberg. Merle Saferstein, who is an honorary member of our family and a prominent author, read every chapter and gave great advice.

My career and my life path have been molded by the outstanding mentorship of the neurosurgery faculty members who trained me. I truly feel as though I stand on the shoulders of giants. As a medical student at Johns Hopkins, I was so fortunate to work in the laboratory of Henry Brem, M.D., whose immense talents are matched only by his kindness and generosity to the hundreds of students he has taken under his wing. Donlin Long, M.D.

(deceased), former chairman of neurosurgery, and Reid Thompson, M.D., who was chief neurosurgery resident at the time, made my experiences as a medical student so meaningful that I chose neurosurgery as a career. Thank you from the bottom of my heart for being nice to the least important person you encountered and altering my life's trajectory.

I had the great privilege of training under the most incredible faculty at Weill Cornell/New York Presbyterian Hospital and Memorial Sloan Kettering Cancer Center. My heartfelt thanks goes to the following faculty for teaching me the nuances of neurosurgery and for your great mentorship: Philip Stieg, M.D., PhD; Philip Gutin, M.D.; Richard Fraser, M.D. (deceased); Mark Bilsky, M.D.; Francis Gamache, M.D.; Eric Holland, M.D.; Michael Kaplitt, M.D., PhD; Michael Lavyne, M.D.; Howard Riina, M.D.; Ted Schwartz, M.D.; Robert Snow, M.D.; and Viviane Tabar, M.D. There are not enough words for me to adequately thank Mark Souweidane, M.D., who is the reason I became a pediatric neurosurgeon. Mark, you are a teacher, mentor, big brother, and best friend and the single greatest influence in my life outside of my immediate family. I can never repay you for all you have done for me.

For my pediatric neurosurgery fellowship at Children's Hospital Los Angeles, I had the great fortune of learning from two incredible pediatric neurosurgeons, J. Gordon McComb, M.D., and Mark Krieger, M.D. Drs. McComb and Krieger, thanks for your example of hard work and dedication and for all the skills you taught me that I still use in the operating room twenty years later.

I have had the great honor of working with and learning from incredible pediatric neurosurgery partners, first in Miami and now in Houston. My heartfelt thanks to Glenn Morrison, M.D.; John Ragheb, M.D.; Sanjiv Bhatia, M.D. (deceased); Greg Olavarria, M.D.; Stephen Fletcher, DO; Manish Shah, M.D.; and Peter Yang, M.D. Pediatric neurosurgery is a team endeavor, and it takes great teamwork to provide optimal care to patients. I am profoundly grateful every day to our incredible physician assistants, Sarah Hubert, PA-C; Eugenia Kelly, PA-C; Emilie Martinez, PA-C; and Anmol Sadruddin, PA-C. I am grateful also to team members Reyna Balderaz, Vianey Blakely, Anne Crocker, Kim Edmonson, Dayeli Frias, Laura Gonzalez, Diana Hernandez, Christine Hill, Marcia Kerr, Paula Maldonado, Alisse Pratt, Sierra Romero-Hearrell, Rose Samaniego, and Bangning Yu. I also want to thank Dick Bassett from the bottom of my heart both for his friendship and for his immense support both for my career and for neurosurgeons in low- and middle-income countries.

Finally, my greatest gratitude is to my wonderful family. My father, Joel Sandberg, M.D., is my inspiration for becoming a doctor, my role model, and hero. My mother, Adele Sandberg, is also my role model and hero for teaching by example how to lead a life of service to others. Mom and Dad, your love and support have been constants in my life that have made my dreams become reality. My sisters, Sheryl and Michelle Sandberg, inspire me with their accomplishments and with their devotion to making the world a better place. Sheryl and Michelle, for my whole life I have counted on your love and support, and you have both enriched my life in so many ways. I also want to thank my wonderful in-laws, Dave Goldberg (deceased), Tom Bernthal, Marc Bodnick, Joe Schefler, Elizabeth Schefler, Ken Schefler, and Sharon Shoham for their love and support over the years.

I have been blessed with the two most amazing children in the whole world. Dalia and Benjamin, thank you for your boundless love and encouragement. In many ways, this book is written for you. You both bring me immeasurable joy, and I am so proud of the extraordinary young woman and man you are growing up to be. And last, my beloved wife, Amy Schefler, M.D. Amy, you have lived through practically every moment of my neurosurgery career. You were with me through the residency years and stayed with me despite getting woken up by countless phone calls night after night. You are my daily sounding board for any struggles I face. You celebrate my successes, and you are there for me on the hard days whether I want to talk or keep things bottled up inside. Everything that I have shared on these pages, and everything that is not on these pages, is more meaningful because of you. I love you with all my heart.

Notes

1: When the Brain Humbles You: Facing Unpredictable Outcomes

1   N. A. Christakis, E. B. Lamont, *British Medical Journal*, 2000;
     320 (7233): 469–72.

2: A Tough Road: The Making of a Pediatric Neurosurgeon

1   Mansukhani, M. P., et al., *Postgraduate Medicine*, 2012; 124
     (4): 241–9.
2   J. L. Denson, et al., *American Journal of Medicine*, 2015; (9):
     994–1000.

3: Hearing the Unthinkable: Helping Families Process a Fatal Diagnosis

1   Harriet Sarnoff Schiff, *The Bereaved Parent* (New York:
     Penguin, 1977).
2   Reiko Schwab, "A Child's Death and Divorce: Dispelling
     the Myth." *Death Studies*; Abington, Vol. 22, Issue 5; 1998:
     445–468.

4: The Greatest Reward: Saving the Life of a Child

1   Talmud (Sanhedrin 37A).

5: Coping with Complications: When the Patient Is Worse after Surgery

1   L. M. Blok, et al., *Journal of Neurosurgery*, 2016; 18 (3): 363–71.
2   J. M. Drake, et al., *Journal of Neurosurgery: Pediatrics*, 2010; 5
     (6): 544–8.
3   C. J. Larkin, et al., *Neurosurgical Focus*, 2020; 49 (5): 15.
4   R. Thomas, et al., *World Neurosurgery*, 2018; 110: 552–559.

7: Bicycles, Bullets, and Beaten Babies: Keeping Our Children Safe

1   J. Olivier, P. Creighton, *American Journal of Epidemiology*, 46 (2017): 278–292.

2   A. O. Asemota, et al., *Journal of Neurotrauma*, 30 (2013): 67–75.

3   US Club Soccer website (usclubsoccer.org).

4   A. C. McKee, et al., *JAMA Neurology*, 80 (2023): 1030–1050.

5   J. W. Brewer Jr., et al., *Journal of Pediatric Surgery*, 54 (2019): 783–791.

6   A. Ianelli, G. Lupi, *Pediatric Neurosurgery*, 41 (2005): 41–45.

About the Author

David I. Sandberg, M.D., is professor and chief of the Division of Pediatric Neurosurgery at McGovern Medical School at UTHealth and Children's Memorial Hermann Hospital in Houston, Texas. He holds the Dr. Marnie Rose Professorship in Pediatric Neurosurgery and the THINK Neurology Chair in Pediatric Tumor Research and Innovation. He serves as codirector of the Pediatric Brain Tumor Program at MD Anderson Children's Cancer Hospital. A magna cum laude graduate of Harvard University, Dr. Sandberg received his medical degree at the Johns Hopkins University School of Medicine. He completed neurosurgery residency training at the Weill Medical College of Cornell University/New York Presbyterian Hospital and Memorial Sloan Kettering Cancer Center. He then completed pediatric neurosurgery fellowship training at Children's Hospital Los Angeles. In 2019, Dr. Sandberg was awarded the Humanitarian Award from the American Association of Neurological Surgeons—one of the highest honors bestowed by that organization. He lives in Houston, Texas, with his wife and two children.